The Bipolar Diet:

Managing Mood, Food and Weight

The Bipolar Diet:

Managing Mood, Food and Weight

By Sarah Freeman

ISBN 978-0-557-20377-2

Disclaimer

This book is offered for informational purposes only and is NOT a substitute for medical advice.

Although we make every effort to offer only accurate information, we cannot guarantee that the information we make available is always correct or current.

Neither Sarah Freeman nor Castlemore LLC warrant or make any representations as to the quality, content, accuracy, or completeness of the information, text, graphics, links and other items contained in this book. Consequently, no one should rely upon any information contained herein, nor make any decisions or take any action based on such information. Consult your doctor before starting any diet or exercise program.

Sarah Freeman and Castlemore LLC are not responsible for any action taken in reliance on the information contained herein and for any damages incurred, whether directly or indirectly, as a result of errors, omissions or discrepancies contained herein.

Contents

Chapter 1: Getting Started: Food and Mood 1

Calm energy 3
How to use this book 5
About me 5

Chapter 2: Bipolar Super Foods 7

1. Coldwater fish 7
2. Lean poultry (fowl) 9
3. Lean red meat 11
4. Egg whites 13
5. High fiber green vegetables 14
6. Berries 15
7. Avocados 15
8. Olive oil 17
9. Water, green tea and herbal tea 19

Chapter 3: The Dirty Dozen: 23

The 12 Worst Foods That Bipolar People Should Almost Never Eat 23

1. Heavily sweetened breakfast cereals 24
2. Soda, "fruit" drinks, soft drinks, flavored coffees 29
3. Sweets, candy, and other refined sugar 30
4. Jellies, jams and preserves 30
5. White bread 30
6. Saturated fats and trans fats 31
7. Ice cream 33
8. Salad dressing 34
9. Potato chips, corn chips, pretzels, and "snack" foods in general 35
10. Cookies, muffins, cakes, pies ... and sorry ... donuts. 36
11. Fast food 37

Chapter 4: Is Your Medication Making You Fat? 43

Which meds are most likely to cause weight gain? 45
Talking to your doctor 46

Fending off the fat 47
Finding the balance... 48

Chapter 5: The Bipolar Thyroid Connection 49

Common thyroid dysfunction symptoms..................... 50
What is an "under-active" thyroid? 51

Chapter 6: Supplements for Bipolar?.........................55

5-HTP 57
Choline 58
Folic acid 58
GABA... 59
Inositol 60
Magnesium 60
Multivitamin and mineral supplements 61
Omega-3 (fish oil) 62
SAMe 64
St. John's Wort 64
Taurine 65
Tyrosine.. 65
Vitamin B12... 66
Vitamin C 67
Zinc... 68

Chapter 7: Winning Strategies: Portions & Planning .69

Portion Control: The basics 71
Visual cues for portion sizes 72
Meal Planning: How much should you eat? 74
How much should I weigh? 75
How much body fat? 77
Managing weight vs managing body fat 77
Calculating your daily calorie requirements.................. 79

Chapter 8: Sample Daily Food Plans 85

Guiding principles 85
To maintain weight.. 86
To lose weight... 87
The starvation response 87
Rules for cutting calories 88

To gain weight 89
1200 calorie plan 90
1400 calorie plan 91
1800 calorie plan 92
2000 calorie plan 94

Alternative 2000 calorie plan 95

Snack Chart & Custom Menu Planner 97

Chapter 9: The Truth About Exercise 101

The benefits of exercise 102
What type of exercise? 103
How much exercise? 104
OK – but I REALLY HATE to exercise 105

Chapter 10: Staying Motivated 107

Baby steps 108
Carrot and stick 108
Get a buddy 109
Avoiding sabotage 109
Kick excuses to the curb 110
Have a little faith 111
Effective goal setting 112

Sources and Further Information 113

**Bonus 1: Special Report on Diabetes and Bipolar
Disorder 117**

Bonus 2: Top 6 Techniques for Managing Moods 123

Bonus 3: Bipolar Diet Glossary 137

Chapter 1:
Getting Started: Food and Mood

Is there a connection between food and mood? You bet there is!

For people with bipolar disorder, this connection is particularly important. We tend to have heightened sensitivity to unhealthy foods such as refined carbohydrates and saturated fats, and the more we eat these unwholesome foods, the more frequent and severe will be the mood swings that result.

Three things you need to know:

1. Dr Fred Goodwin and Dr Kay Redfield Jamison have documented a pattern of reactive hypoglycemia in people with bipolar disorder. Reactive hypoglycemia is low blood sugar that occurs 1-3 hours after a meal. The symptoms include fatigue, depression, anxiety, irritability, craving sweets, poor concentration and confusion, panic attacks, clumsiness, pounding or racing heart, numbness or coldness in the extremities, and outburst of rage. (You can read more about this in Chapter 3.) **The solution? Eat in a way that stabilizes insulin and blood sugar as much as possible!**

2. A 2009 study showed that people with bipolar disorder are 1.5 - 2 times more likely to die from physical diseases such as heart disease, stroke, and diabetes than are members of the general population. Heart disease, hypertension and

diabetes are all at epidemic proportions in developed countries like the US anyway. **For people with bipolar disorder, it is twice as urgent to follow a food and exercise plan that will manage these risks!**

3. Research has shown that people with bipolar disorder tend to be more likely than other members of the public to suffer from deficiencies in omega-3 fatty acids, vitamin B12, folic acid, and vitamin C. **It is easy to adjust your diet so that you consume more of these critical nutrients, or obtain them from an affordable daily multivitamin.**

The 3 goals of *The Bipolar Diet* are directly tied to critical research findings:

1. Minimize mood swings through stabilizing blood sugar and insulin response.

2. Protect against heart disease, stroke, diabetes and other physical diseases that particularly "target" people with bipolar disorder.

3. Control weight, especially for the many people that have gained weight due to their bipolar medications.

Over 35% of people with bipolar disorder are obese. This is the highest percentage for any psychiatric illness. However, it is possible for all people with bipolar disorder to maintain a healthy height, and even to improve overall physical as well as mental health. This is *The Bipolar Diet* mission.

How did I discover the principles of *The Bipolar Diet*? After gaining over 40 lbs from meds like:

- Lexapro (made me manic and fat)

- Neurontin (didn't work and made me fat)
- Depakote (I cried all day, my hair fell out, and yep, made me fat)
- Lithium (for me, the best of a bad lot, but everyone is different)

I started researching the connections between diet and bipolar disorder.

My goal was to discover nutritional strategies that would support stable moods while enabling me to manage my weight. My quest led me to the principles of calm energy, and to the writing of this book.

Calm energy

The first time I encountered the phrase "calm energy" I had a true light bulb moment. Wouldn't it be wonderful to have energy and vigor, but no mania? Wouldn't it be great to feel peaceful and relaxed, without sliding down into depression? Calm energy sounded perfect. A way to enjoy a bright, energized mood, without the rollercoaster of mood swings, rapid cycling, or mixed states. I had to learn more . . .

Calm Energy is the title of a book by mood scientist, Robert Thayer. It explains how people are able to regulate their moods through food and exercise. In particular, the book explains:

- How rising stress levels underlie our current obesity epidemic.
- Our tendency, whether bipolar or not, to self-medicate through food.
- The scientific underpinnings of the food/mood connection.

For many of us, our usual state is a combination of tense and tired. "Calm energy" is that sweet spot where we experience the perfect balance of relaxation and energy, achieved through optimizing our body chemistry through sensible eating and physical activity.

It is similar to the concept of "the zone", described by Dr Barry Sears:

> *"The Zone is not some mystical place or some clever marketing term. It is a real physiological state in your body that is not too high, but not too low. This requires treating food as if it were a drug to be taken at the right dose and at the right time. Your diet affects hormones that are hundreds of times more powerful than any drug. In many respects, food will be the most powerful drug you will ever take because you are using this drug at least three times a day for the rest of your life. Thus your diet can be your greatest ally or worst enemy."*

The Depression and Bipolar Support Alliance (DBSA) has also studied the food/mood connection.

DBSA advises people with bipolar disorder that they may benefit even more than members of the general population from adopting sound nutritional practices that:

- provide the correct balance of protein and carbs, and

- provide proper quantities of vitamins, amino acids, fatty acids, minerals, and fiber.

The Bipolar Diet conforms to the DBSA guidelines, but gives you a lot more information so you can construct a detailed and customized plan that is perfect for you.

How to use this book

Ideally read it slowly and carefully from beginning to end ☺

If you are pressed for time, or have a different learning style, I suggest the following:

- Please read *Chapter 2: Bipolar Super Foods and Chapter 3: The Dirty Dozen*, as it is easier to customize and follow the meal plans if you understand why certain foods are particularly "good" for people with bipolar, whereas others are definitely bad choices.

- The most detailed chapter is *Chapter 7: Portions and Planning*. Don't skip over this. It has essential information for calculating your ideal body weight, body fat %, and how many calories a day you, as an individual, need in order to lose, gain or maintain body fat.

And remember: There are NO nutritional supplements or dietary plans that a consensus of experts judge as having been proven effective (by themselves) in the treatment of any serious mental illness, including bipolar disorder.

The Bipolar Diet can lessen the severity and frequency of mood swings, improve your overall physical and mental health, and alleviate some symptoms of bipolar disorder. It will NOT cure bipolar disorder and is intended to be used as an enhancement to your professional medical care – NOT a replacement!

About me

Like many people with bipolar disorder, my diagnosis came relatively late in life, after a burst of manic craziness that turned my pretty much perfect life into a train wreck.

You can read the whole torrid tale in the About Me section of my Bipolar Lives website at www.bipolar-lives.com.

Today my life is back on track. In fact, it is wonderful.

I have learned my lessons about food and mood the hard way - and the weight gain from my medications was a nightmare!

Everything I talk about in this book is based on clinical research which I then applied to myself. It is this combination of scientific evidence - tested again through my own personal experience - that makes me so confident of the results.

Diet and exercise are an essential part of my wellness plan. I will follow *The Bipolar Diet* for the rest of my life. Please join me in the way of calm energy.

Chapter 2:
Bipolar Super Foods

1. Coldwater fish

Why so much fuss about fish? Quite simply, fish is pure brain food. In particular, coldwater or "fatty" fish such as salmon, sardines and mackerel are especially high in omega-3 fatty acids. Research shows these are crucial for optimal brain regulation and brain chemistry.

The essential fats in fish oil that are most important for brain health are eicosapentaenic acid (EPA) and docosahexaenoic acid (DHA).

Approximately 50% of the brain is fat, and "good" fats play a much more vital role in brain chemistry than many of us realize. Making sure that 50% of the brain is being primed with good fats such as the EPA and DHA from fish, instead of unhealthy fats such as the saturated fats in fast food, has a profound effect on brain chemistry. For example DHA does everything from regulating the release of feel good chemicals like serotonin, to transporting nutrients into brain cells, and efficiently removing the brain's cellular waste.

Some other compounds in the brain that need DHA for proper regulation are:

- prostaglandins (which control many other hormones, which is probably why fish oil has been found to relieve PMS),

- leukotrienes (which are involved in allergic reactions and inflammatory responses in the body), and

- cytokines (which play a role in autoimmune disorders and inflammation. The presence of pro-inflammatory cytokines has been linked to both bipolar depression and mania).

Of course today there is a lot more awareness of the importance of omegas for everyone – we see omega fortified products in every aisle of the grocery store - eggs, cereals, spreads – even sodas. Most people will definitely improve their health and well-being by regularly consuming these important nutrients. However, the health benefits of fish and omega-3 fatty acids are especially significant for someone living with bipolar disorder:

1. Research has shown a direct link between deficiency in the essential fatty acids and bipolar disorder.

2. Research has also shown that increased consumption relieves both depressive and manic symptoms – the holy grail of any bipolar treatment.

3. Many people with bipolar disorder also have ADHD-type difficulties such as "foggy thinking" or racing thoughts. Research shows that people who eat fish regularly have better cognitive, learning, and memory skills. Studies in children also support this. Boys aged 6-12 with low levels of omega-3s have more learning problems, temper tantrums, sleep problems and behavior problems.

In summary, eating coldwater fish may strike directly at a potential cause of bipolar and will help prevent mood swings in either direction. A fish rich diet will also support overall brain function, leading to clearer thinking.

Eating fish regularly can be especially helpful for young people where there is confusion over whether the diagnosis should be a mood disorder, an attention deficit disorder, a conduct disorder, or even all three.

The clinical evidence and the benefits shown in these studies are discussed in more detail on the Bipolar Lives website – see Fish Oil Benefits at www.bipolar-lives.com/fish-oil-benefits.html.

(Don't like fish? See *Chapter 6: Supplements for Bipolar?*)

2. Lean poultry (fowl)

What do I mean by "lean poultry"? The number one foods in this category are chicken breast and turkey breast. We are talking about real, whole foods here – not processed luncheon meats, and "lean" means with the skin off and grilled, baked, or broiled - definitely NOT fried chicken.

There are many arguments to support a diet based on the sort of lean protein – small wild game – that humanity has evolved on. Our ancient ancestors ate a natural diet based on the lifestyle of a hunter gatherer, and our brains, digestive systems, and hormonal systems all function best when we feed our bodies the foods we were designed for.

Protein is especially important for people with bipolar disorder because of the role it plays in stabilizing blood sugar. Stable blood sugar will minimize mood swings and provide you with the kind of steady, calm energy that you need. Not sluggish, and not hyper. Just as with your medication, you are searching for that "sweet spot" – think of it as a Goldilocks food – your diet is a critical tool in supporting you to feel "just right" – not too much of this, or that.

Protein also has the advantage of making you feel fuller, faster. Research shows that people who eat protein as part of every meal tend to eat less overall. Eating enough protein is a key factor in appetite control and will reduce the amount of food you eat afterward.

Many nutritionists have struggled to understand why high protein, low carb diets are so successful for weight loss when they fly in the face of what, for many years, was accepted as the conventional wisdom, embodied in the traditional, carb-heavy, food pyramid. The answer is that eating more protein is more satisfying and leads to lower overall calorie consumption. Further, even though protein foods often contain fat, because people on high protein diets eat less overall, they are not consuming dangerously high amounts of fat, as was once feared. Of course, by eating LEAN protein, you get the best of both worlds – more satisfaction per fewer calories consumed, while avoiding too many animal fats which can be dangerous for the heart.

Protein is also considered a Bipolar Super Food because it supplies the nutrients that act as the building blocks for neurotransmitters. Lean chicken and turkey are excellent sources of L-tryptophan, L-tyrosine, and GABA:

- L-tryptophan increases serotonin in the brain and is a safe, effective natural sleep aid. It is also considered to have antidepressant qualities.

- L-tyrosine is needed for the brain's production of the "feel good" chemicals dopamine and norepinephrine.

Research shows that as a supplement it has no apparent benefit for those who currently enjoy good physical and mental health. However, it does boost mood and cognitive performance for individuals who are suffering from stress.

- GABA is an important amino acid that regulates our excitability. With too little GABA we become over-stimulated and/or anxious. Bipolar patients often show low levels of GABA in the bloodstream. We need GABA in order to relax and sleep properly, and in order for our brains to exercise appropriate impulse control. It is best to get GABA from food, instead of supplements. (See Chapter 6.)

3. Lean red meat

Lean red meat offers all the protein advantages discussed above for lean chicken or turkey. In addition, red meat is high in vitamin B12, iron, zinc, and creatine. Anyone who has a mood disorder needs to ensure they are consuming an abundance of B12, and educate themselves on the importance of this critical nutrient.

Vitamin B12 is normally involved in the metabolism of every cell of the body. Vitamin B12 deficiency can potentially cause severe and irreversible damage, especially to the brain and nervous system. At levels only slightly lower than normal, a range of symptoms such as fatigue, depression, and poor memory may be experienced.

Studies have shown that both mania and depression may be associated with vitamin B12 deficiency, and that these symptoms cleared after the subjects took B12 supplementation. This does not mean that all bipolar results from B12 deficiency, or that all bipolar can be cured by taking enough B12. Rather, as with all the nutritional relationships we describe, following *The Bipolar Diet* reduces any symptoms that are related to poor nutrition, and fortifies you against unnecessary mood swings and other symptoms.

Many menstruating women fail to get enough dietary iron and as a result become anemic. Iron-deficiency anemia causes symptoms such as inattention and slowed cognitive processes, and which often look a lot like some of the signs of ADHD and/or bipolar disorder. Having a diet with an adequate amount of iron prevents anemia and the associated symptoms. This improves overall health and quality of life, and also reduces the chances of a misdiagnosis. Although far more common in women, dietary related anemia can also be a problem for men. Vitamin deficiency anemia may occur when vitamin B12 and folic acid are deficient as both of these are needed to make red blood cells. All good reasons to include lean red meat as a dietary staple!

Creatine is mainly popular as a sports supplement because it can help build muscle mass. However, it also boosts cognitive performance and has neuro-protective properties and is therefore of definite benefit to the bipolar brain.

Today there are many red meat products tailored to people who follow a low fat diet. The suggestion to eat lean red meat is not a blank check encouraging you to eat large amounts of unhealthy animal fats. Instead, buy the leanest cuts you can find, and always control portion size. The difference is significant. A large one pound plus restaurant steak could have 100 grams of fat. However, 6 ounces of lean, trimmed top round steak (our suggested portion size) has only 9 grams of fat. This increases to a much more significant 37 grams of fat for a 6 ounce untrimmed porterhouse.

4. Egg whites

Egg whites may well be the perfect protein.

For vegetarians or those who dislike eating red meat and/or fish, or who have reason to follow a very low fat diet, egg whites deliver a flexible alternative.

Heaps of protein and no unhealthy fats – almost sounds too good to be true, doesn't it?

Also, egg whites come in a variety of forms – you can buy fresh eggs and separate out the yolks, buy Egg Beaters or an organic alternative, and even egg white protein powder. (I buy a chocolate flavored one for shakes and smoothies – a life saver if you are in a hurry or watching calories.)

Along with the all important protein, egg whites are good sources of other nutrients that help stabilize and brighten moods so that you feel happy but calm – not manic. They contain vital mood nutrients such as B12, folate (folic acid), iron and vitamin D, as well as minerals such as magnesium and zinc.

In terms of weight management, egg whites really are the ideal food. As Tom Venuto, a leading fat-loss guru has explained in his brilliant weight loss manual, *Burn the Fat, Feed the Muscle:*

> *"The name of the game in fat-burning, muscle-building nutrition is to eat a lean protein with every meal. With zero fat, egg whites are as lean as lean proteins get. Egg whites are right up there with chicken breasts as one of the top three*

lean proteins of choice for losing fat and gaining muscle."

As well as my beloved chocolate protein powder, I use the organic version of Egg Beaters, available from Publix, and separate my fresh eggs using a ratio of 1:3, meaning I keep one yolk in every three eggs when I want scrambled eggs or an extra yummy weekend omelet.

5. High fiber green vegetables

Mom was right! You really do need to eat plenty of broccoli, spinach, green beans, and other green veggies with plenty of fiber to have true mental and physical health.

In terms of weight management and avoiding the physical health complications that often accompany bipolar disorder, including heart disease, stroke, and diabetes, eating your veggies is pretty well a no brainer.

How about the mood benefits?

The high fiber of these green super foods will prevent mood swings by stabilizing blood sugar. There is also a link between mood and regularity. That's right! When we joke about sour or grumpy faced people looking constipated, we may be literally correct. Researchers have discovered a statistically significant link between constipation and depression. Getting regular will make you feel both physically and mentally lighter.

The most important mood nutrients from green vegetables are folic acid, iron, calcium, B-vitamins, and the stress busting vitamin C.

Spinach is a great example of a classic happy food that can elevate mood safely with no danger of inducing mania. As well as iron, it is packed with folic acid that is essential for producing enough serotonin for a "feel-good" brain. Folic acid is right up there with omega-3s in terms of a wealth of credible scientific evidence that it is as powerful as medication in relieving depression. We will talk about folic acid in more detail later, but in the meantime, please eat your vegetables!

6. Berries

The ideal bipolar diet places special emphasis on blueberries, raspberries, cherries, and cranberries.

As well as being packed with antioxidants to stave off free-radical damage, cancer and protect your physical health, these berries can promote clearer thinking and have many neuro-protective qualities.

They are a healthy way of getting the carbs and sweet tastes that many people with bipolar crave, without sending your blood sugar and your moods off on a roller coaster. Instead of sugar, which basically makes people crazy and has no nutritional value, berries are full neuro-nutrients to nourish your brain and assist brain chemistry.

7. Avocados

Avocados are a great fresh food that can be eaten raw and make a perfect snack.

What are the general nutritional benefits of avocados?

Avocados contain the healthy monounsaturated fat oleic acid, and have been shown in studies to both lower "bad" LDL cholesterol and raise "good" HDL cholesterol.

Avocados are also high in potassium – a mineral that promotes heart health, lowers blood pressure, and can even protect against stroke. Oleic acid has been shown to help keep women safe from breast cancer. There is something for the boys as well – avocados also contain the carotenoids lutein, zeaxanthin, alpha-carotene and beta-carotene, plus significant quantities of tocopherols (vitamin E) – a combination shown to inhibit the growth of prostate cancer cells.

These protective qualities in relation to heart health, blood pressure, stroke, and cancer are important for people with bipolar disorder. Recent studies have found bipolar disorder increases the risk of early death from medical illnesses, particularly heart disease, respiratory disease, stroke, and diabetes.

Avocados are also packed with vitamin K, vitamin B6, vitamin C, vitamin A, vitamin D, omega 6, folate and copper. They also have the highest dietary fiber of any fruit.

Avocados are also protective of the liver and eating avocado is usually a cornerstone of any liver cleansing or liver regeneration diet. Liver health is crucial for effective fat and sugar metabolism, weight control, and healthy digestion.

There are 3 main reasons why avocados are included in our list of Bipolar Super Foods:

1. Avocado is a wonderful source of folate. Folate (folic acid) is an essential neuronutrient, yet 75% Americans are deficient in it. However, folate is key to maintaining good moods and is discussed in detail in *Chapter 6: Supplements for Bipolar?* Folate/folic acid has been linked to bipolar disorder, and is one of the few supplements that

has been proven to be beneficial specifically for bipolar people. Importantly, deficiency in folic acid has been associated with both depression and mania.

2. The very high monounsaturated "good" fat content keeps the receptors in your brain sensitive to serotonin, which helps combat bipolar depression.

3. Avocados are a very versatile, satisfying, and portable snack. It may sound strange to be emphasizing the value of a food based on logistical factors. However, sometimes utilitarian features can be "make or break". For people who are stressed, time poor, and adjusting to major lifestyle changes, finding healthy snacks that are convenient and easy to prepare greatly increases the likelihood of sticking to smart food choices. The goal of mood stabilization is much easier to reach with stable blood sugar, and steady, calm energy. Regular healthy snacks are a must.

8. Olive oil

In ancient Greece olive oil was known as "liquid gold".

Throughout this book there are many mentions of "good fats" versus "bad fats". Understand the distinction, change your diet accordingly, and you will find this one simple substitution can dramatically increase your physical and mental health.

There is scientific evidence suggesting that eating about 2 tablespoons of olive oil daily may reduce the risk of heart disease as olive oil contains monounsaturated fat. However, PLEASE REMEMBER, to achieve this benefit, you MUST use olive oil to REPLACE a similar amount of unhealthy saturated fat (for example butter), and NOT increase the total number of calories you eat in a day.

One of the most healthful aspects of olive oil is the high content of oleic acid, which boosts memory and reduces blood pressure.

Olive oil also assists cholesterol regulation, and is a powerful anti-inflammatory agent.

Another important benefit of olive oil is its ability to displace omega-6 fats, while not having any impact on omega-3 fats. In this way, olive oil builds a healthier balance between omega-6 fats and omega-3 fats, making you happier and smarter.

It seems counter intuitive, but olive oil also helps weight loss. Many people with bipolar struggle with weight gain. Research shows that overweight people who add olive oil to their diet are more likely to slash pounds. This is thought to be because the rich, fulfilling taste and texture of olive oil delivers "more bang for the buck" and leads to lower fat and calorie consumption overall.

As stated previously, people with bipolar disorder experience higher than usual death rates from obesity related conditions, heart disease and stroke, so preventative strategies are even more critical for us than for the population at large.

It is the anti-inflammatory properties of olive oil that are of particular interest though. Stress triggers inflammation throughout the body, including the brain and the gut. This inflammation compromises our gut's ability to absorb critical neuro-nutrients, and our brain's ability to regulate mood.

These anti-inflammatory qualities also help reduce aches and pains such as headaches and even the pain from arthritis.

9. Water, green tea and herbal tea

This book talks a lot about all the things people with bipolar disorder should not drink, or should drink only in moderation - sodas, coffee, alcohol – even milk. However, please don't think that water and teas are being suggested only because there is nothing else left to drink!

In living with bipolar we must be constantly striving to eliminate the negatives and accentuate the positives. Water and herbal teas offer distinct heath benefits to support calm, sustained energy and bright moods, without fueling dangerous mood swings.

Consider the following:

- Water rids your body of toxins and waste products. It will help your meds work better, lessen side effects, and control weight. Most importantly, it will boost energy without the risk of mania or irritability. It will also reduce bloating and other PMS discomfort – important as women with bipolar tend to experience more severe PMS symptoms. Sometimes cravings for sugar are really signs of dehydration, so try drinking two glasses of water instead. Weight gain and mood swings from sugar and other "bad" carbs are the enemy. Try drowning them with H2O – the single most important nutrient your body needs.

- Rooibos or Red Bush tea has powerful antioxidant benefits, but unlike green tea it does not contain caffeine. This is a wonderful drink that is refreshing yet relaxing.

- Chamomile tea is a natural sleep aid – start drinking it in the late afternoon/early evening instead of immediately before bed so you don't defeat the purpose by having to wake up to use the bathroom. This natural relaxant is a much better choice than caffeine, given the links between bipolar disorder and sleep.

- Green tea does contain caffeine (although decaf versions are available – my own favorite drink) but is much healthier than coffee and assists in losing weight and fighting depression. The amino acid L-theanine, found almost exclusively in the tea plant, actively alters the attention networks of the brain, according to results of human trials announced in September 2007. It has been proposed that theanine is absorbed by the small intestine and crosses the blood-brain barrier, where it affects the brain's neurotransmitters and increases alpha brain-wave activity. The result is a calmer, yet more alert, state of mind.

Use the ancient ritual of taking time to prepare and serve and savor your tea. Set routines and regular downtime are hugely beneficial just in themselves.

Be careful of some herbal teas – they can clash with medication or have unwanted side effects, especially if you are pregnant or in the throes of a serious mood episode. Stick with the ones listed here unless you have a personal favorite that you KNOW is safe. Also be cautious of diuretic teas. They often don't lead to genuine weight loss and may actually contribute to dehydration.

Of course for all people, regardless of their mental or emotional health, adequate hydration is essential to life. Many people are dehydrated without even realizing it. The symptoms of the sort of constant low-level dehydration that is common today include irritability and fatigue – easy to dismiss as part of a mood disorder or as medication side effects.

Try to follow the 8 glasses a day rule of thumb as a minimum, and monitor urination. If you are drinking enough you will need to empty your bladder every 3-5 hours, and your urine will be pale or almost colorless. If you need to use the bathroom more infrequently or have dark urine, these are worrying signs that your body needs more fluid.

(Some bipolar medications such as lithium require a delicate balance of not too much and not too little fluid intake, and may have frequent urination as an unwanted side effect. You can find out more about this on the Bipolar Lives website in our Lithium section at http://www.bipolar-lives.com/lithium.html.)

Chapter 3: The Dirty Dozen:

The 12 Worst Foods That Bipolar People Should Almost Never Eat

What we are doing in Chapter 2 and Chapter 3 (this chapter) is giving you an "eat this, not that" blueprint that you can use so to make informed, empowering food choices that will help balance your moods, instead of aggravating the manic depressive roller coaster. By using these guidelines to figure out what you SHOULD eat – as well as what you should NOT eat – you can choose foods that will have a positive impact on your moods and brain chemistry.

Then, depending on your goals, you can focus on building a deep reservoir of "calm energy", and on losing, gaining or maintaining weight, depending on where you are at right now. By learning to choose the "Bipolar Super Foods" instead of the "Dirty Dozen" as the foundation of your diet, you can construct a free-form eating plan based on your own personal needs and preferences, or you can follow one of the food plans laid out for you in Chapter 8. (In *Chapter 8: Sample Daily Food Plans,* the food plans are low calorie and are of particular interest if your goal is weight loss.)

The "Dirty Dozen" are those foods that I would like to see you avoid as much as is humanly possible. What makes a food a candidate for the Dirty Dozen? Key characteristics include:

- Likely to cause dramatics spikes and dips in blood sugar and encourage mood swings.

- Proven negative effect on brain chemistry.

- Empty calories with low nutritional value so that all you are doing is gaining weight with no contribution to nourishing your brain or your body.

- Proven triggers that will worsen mood swings and contribute to addictive, "self-medicating" cycles of counter-productive eating.

- Proven negative physiological effects such as leaching your body of minerals, vitamins, and crucial neuro-nutrients.

- Lots of unhealthy saturated and trans fats, contributing to the tendency for people with bipolar disorder to suffer higher than normal rates of heart disease, stroke, diabetes and other preventable disease.

It would be impractical and unrealistic to say NEVER eat ANY of these foods. After all, I can practically guarantee that some of your favorites will be included here – I know mine are ☺

However, what I AM saying is AVOID these as much as you can, and plan your eating so that you indulge in these just once or twice a week. Don't worry for now if this sounds challenging – in Chapter 7 and Chapter 10 you will learn exactly how to do this so that you don't feel deprived and no super-human discipline is required.

1. Heavily sweetened breakfast cereals

It is hard to imagine anything more self-sabotaging for a person with a mood disorder than to start their day with a cocktail of refined sugar and assorted other simple carbohydrates. Stable blood sugar greatly increases the likelihood of stable moods, calm energy, and clear thinking.

Breakfast cereal is the most advertised product in America, and probably the most toxic. Don't be fooled by the billions of dollars of crazy claims being made to persuade you to buy the ultimate empty calories. The science in favor of a protein and complex carb start to your day is overwhelming.

A major premise of *The Bipolar Diet* is that sugar and refined/simple carbohydrates are about the worst things you could eat in terms of both your mental and physical health. **If you get nothing else from this book, please study the following 4 paragraphs carefully** – understand the bipolar/sugar connection (and change your diet accordingly) and you will see a dramatic improvement in your ability to manage or even avoid episodes of mania and depression.

1. The leading medical text on bipolar disorder, *Manic-Depressive Illness: Bipolar Disorders and Recurrent Depression* by Frederick Goodwin and Kay Redfield Jamison, states:

   "Bipolar patients tend to have a pattern of reactive hypoglycemia, in which simple carbohydrates in the morning can produce an excessive increase in blood sugar, followed by an excessive decrease . . . [leading to] feeling tired, fuzzy-headed, or irritable. To relieve these symptoms, patients often ingest more carbohydrates . . . in effect chasing their blood sugar throughout the day . . . and in the process take in many additional calories."

2. What do Drs Goodwin and Jamison mean by "reactive hypoglycemia"? Low blood sugar (hypoglycemia) usually occurs while fasting. But reactive hypoglycemia is low blood sugar that occurs after a meal — usually one to three hours after eating. The symptoms include fatigue, depression, anxiety, irritability, craving sweets, poor concentration and confusion, panic attacks, clumsiness, pounding or racing heart, numbness or coldness in the extremities, and outbursts of rage. Anything sound familiar?

3. There is no way of breaking the link between unstable blood sugar and unstable moods. When your blood sugar spikes, your pancreas goes into insulin overdrive, pumping out insulin in order to convert the excess sugar into stored fat. This rush of insulin causes your blood sugar to plummet, making you tired, angry, and starving for more carbs. Give in and eat more sugar and the whole cycle repeats. There is no getting off the sugar/mood roller coaster. Too much sugar and you feel tired and fuzzy headed. Too little sugar and you feel impatient and aggressive. Your brain requires a relatively low but constant supply of sugar, and the ideal sugar/insulin balance falls within a very narrow range.

4. Bipolar people are especially sensitive, needing even smaller than usual amounts of sugar to set off a hypoglycemic reaction, and experiencing greater than average mood swings as their blood sugar rises and falls. However, instead of getting off the blood sugar roller coaster, folks with bipolar are more likely to "chase" their blood sugar and self-medicate with sweets, snacks, and other "bad" carbs.

If the four points above make sense to you, you will understand why the number one food on my "hit list" is sugary cereals that sabotage your brain chemistry at the very beginning of your day.

The best way to counter this dangerous cycle is to:

- avoid sugar
- eat regular small meals/snacks every 4 hours
- eat plenty of protein
- eat plenty of fiber, and
- stay hydrated.

Is all cereal evil? Not at all! If you MUST have cereal then good choices are traditional oatmeal (not the sweetened instant kind full of artificial ingredients), especially if you mix in a scoop of protein powder, or brands like Kashi and Ezekiel that include nuts, seeds and whole grains. The smart way to enjoy these is to use Hood protein milk and/or natural yoghurt with them to increase the ratio of protein to carbs and overall nutritional value.

The table below lists nutritional values for some of the best and the worst of the better known popular American cereals per serving:

The Bipolar Diet

Cereal	Calories	Trans Fat	Saturated Fat	Total Fat	Protein	Carbs	Sugar	Fiber
Cheerios (General Mills)	100	0g	0g	2g	3g	20g	1g	3g
All Bran Original (Kelloggs)	80	0g	0g	1g	4g	23g	6g	10g
Go Lean (Kashi)	140	0g	0g	1g	13g	30g	6g	10g
Shredded Wheat (Post)	160	0g	0g	1g	5g	37g	0g	6g
Fiber One Original (Post)	60	0g	0g	1g	2g	25g	0g	14g
Special K Protein Plus (Kelloggs)	100	0g	0.5g	3g	10g	14g	2g	5g
Instant Oatmeal Weight Control (Quakers)	160	0g	0.5g	3g	7g	29g	1g	6g
Fruit Loops (Kelloggs)	110	0g	0.5g	1g	1g	25g	12g	1g
Cocoa Puffs (General Mills)	110	0g	0g	1.5g	1g	23g	12g	1g
Raisin Bran (Kelloggs)	190	0g	0g	1.5g	5g	45g	19g	7g
Grape Nuts (Post)	200	0g	0g	1g	6g	48g	4g	7g
Total Whole Grain (General Mills)	100	0g	0g	0.5g	2g	23g	5g	3g

Remember – if you start your day with a jolt of refined sugar and simple carbs you will be on the blood sugar/mood swing roller coaster before you hit your front door. Please study the table above - and the labels on some of your favorite cereals. I LOVE Raisin Bran! However, if you look at the figures above then I am sure you will understand why I am much happier and healthier since swapping to Special K Protein Plus and Go Lean by Kashi.

2. Soda, "fruit" drinks, soft drinks, flavored coffees

We have learned about the predisposition of people with bipolar disorder to hypoglycemia and its devastating heightening of mood swings in both directions, with sugar being the villain of the piece. Suppose I was to also tell you that sugar leaches your body of minerals, many of which are essential "neuro-nutrients" – ingredients necessary for healthy brain chemistry and the production of feel good and mood stabilizing neurotransmitters? My guess is that you are starting to get the message – sugar and bipolar disorder just do not play well together. Imagine then the hazards of LIQUID SUGAR – sugar that you drink IN ADDITION to the sugar that you eat. Research proves that sugary drinks are especially dangerous, as when people consume extra sugar and calories as liquid, they tend NOT to compensate by cutting back on their food intake.

A study from the American Journal of Public Health found that people who drink 2½ cans of soda daily are three times more likely to be depressed and anxious, compared with those who drink fewer. Research into other sweetened drinks would probably yield even worse results, given the high amount of sugar involved. For example, I have included flavored coffee drinks because a Starbucks 24 oz Strawberries & Crème Frappuccino contains 750 calories and 120 grams of sugar.

3. Sweets, candy, and other refined sugar

If breakfast cereals that are 10-50% sugar are toxic for people fighting manic-depressive illness, then how would you describe "mainlining" 100% the real thing? Any "pure" sugar food, such as candies, syrup for your pancakes, or sugar in your coffee is simply empty calories that will play havoc with your moods, energy and overall health but have absolutely no nutritional benefit.

4. Jellies, jams and preserves

"More of the same" or "see above", although there is one added twist. Many of these products promote themselves as diet foods, either because they are sweetened with artificial sweeteners or because they contain no "added" sugar. Do NOT be fooled! The likely consequences for your blood sugar and your moods are still NEGATIVE. Even without "added" cane sugar, these are still blood sugar time-bombs because the fruit sugar from the heavily processed fruit will cause the same spike and crash effect.

5. White bread

White bread is a highly refined simple carbohydrate, and right up there with sugar in terms of the archetypical "bad" carb. Some products are nothing more than empty calories, whereas some are marginally better in that they have been fortified by the manufacturer who may have added back in some fiber or useful nutrients such as vitamins or iron. However, even if there has been a last minute attempt at a nutritional boost through some additives, white bread is another blood sugar and mood saboteur that you are better off without.

6. Saturated fats and trans fats

There are two important reasons to avoid these unhealthy fats. The first is that they damage the brain, disrupt brain chemistry and play havoc with moods, all of which will make your illness worse, when instead you could be consuming "good fats" such as omega-3s which would actually help you.

The second is the overall effect on physical, rather than mental, health. This is relevant in a book about Bipolar Diet because recent research has shown that people with bipolar disorder are more likely to suffer from a variety of deadly physical diseases.

You see, it turns out that being bipolar is a lot like being a smoker. It dramatically increases the risk of early death, especially from heart disease, respiratory diseases, stroke, and diabetes. This research is based on a comprehensive review of 17 studies involving more than 331,000 patients. These studies indicated that the risk of early death from a medical illness was from 35 percent to 200 percent higher for us than for the general population. The picture is scary and depressing and the numbers are truly staggering. However, these are all illnesses that have a strong diet and lifestyle component and some simple preventative strategies can help protect you. It is one of the main themes of this book. *The Bipolar Diet* is designed to stabilize moods, boost moods safely without flipping into mania, AND protect against the heart disease, respiratory disease, stroke and diabetes that stalk people with bipolar disorder.

Today everyone knows that saturated fats and heart disease are tightly linked. However, even though saturated fat should be avoided, very minimal consumption (less that 7% of total calorie intake) is probably safe.

In contrast, trans fats are such major contributors to heart disease that many national, state and local governments are banning their use in restaurants, for example in California and New York. According to health authorities, trans fats have no nutritional value and pose such a serious health risk that there is no safe level of consumption. One major study concluded that *"On a per-calorie basis, trans fats appear to increase the risk of [coronary heart disease] more than any other macronutrient"*.

There is no doubt that saturated fat and trans fat are major contributors to the physical diseases that kill people with bipolar disorder in such frightening and disproportionately high numbers. But what about their effects on mood?

In order for our brains to function properly, they must be lubricated, supple and fluid. Healthy fats such as omega-3s and olive oil are very good for this. However trans fats make brain tissue rigid and inflexible. That is right – they actually alter the cell membranes of the brain. Another problem is that trans fats accumulate in the brain and displace the good fats, especially DHA. The critical neurotransmitter dopamine is depleted, leading to depression and cognitive impairment and decline. In summary, the "bad" fats both damage the brain in their own right, and also decrease the amount of "good" fats in the brain, compounding problems with low moods and foggy thinking. (You can read about this in more detail in *Brain-Building Nutrition* by Michael A. Schmidt.)

As well as having such a negative and direct impact on our brain chemistry, there is also the problem of how "bad" fats can affect insulin. It turns out that "bad" fat, like sugar, causes our bodies to become insulin resistant. Research shows that a diet of more than 37% fat causes insulin resistance. However, the really important findings are that it is the QUALITY and NOT just QUANTITY of fat that matters. When research subjects consumed less than 37% of their daily calories from fat, it was found that saturated fats increase the insulin response, whereas monosaturated fats (such as olive oil) decreased it. Eating healthy fats will protect you from going into "insulin overdrive" which in turn prevents physical problems like diabetes, high blood pressure and obesity, and mental and emotional problems from crashing glucose such as depression, anger, and clouded judgment and thinking. Saturated fats, on the other hand, encourage excess insulin and all the physical and mental health problems that go with it.

7. Ice cream

Ok – we have covered the basics – sugar and "bad" fats are the two "foods" that represent the most serious mental and physical health risks for people with bipolar disorder. Now let's talk about what happens when you put the two together . . .

One particularly seductive sugar/fat combo is ice cream. In fact, ice cream is possibly my favorite food. If I could in good conscience leave it off this list I sure as heck would. Also, my first business was an ice cream stand so I have a special affection for it, and am always fascinated by new ice cream trends, brands, and products. It is also the single fastest way to stack on weight ever invented. In fact, the combination of sugar, fat, and calorie density makes ice cream the ultimate fat storing, blimpifying obesity bomb. In fairness it does contain some calcium, but compare that to all the artificial colors, artificial flavors, preservatives, emulsifiers and stabilizers, and you are talking nutrition hell.

If weight control is one of your goals there are some facts and figures you need to copy down and stick on your freezer door - one cup of regular premium vanilla contains around 350 calories and 20 grams of (mostly saturated) fat. A cup of Haagen Daz Belgian Chocolate has 660 calories and 36 grams of fat.

Now as an ice cream addict I am NOT going to ask the impossible and say never eat it. On my birthday I went to Dairy Queen for a hot chocolate fudge sundae – and because I can't go a whole year without indulging, I sometimes buy the sugar free, low/no fat products – 200 calories that I can burn off with a brisk walk.

8. Salad dressing

Ok – not all salad dressings are bad. It is possible to make a delicious and healthy dressing out of traditional ingredients such as olive oil, lemon juice, Dijon mustard – all kinds of things.

However, the overwhelming majority of restaurant and supermarket salad dressings are VERY unhealthy and really do destroy the whole point of ordering a salad in the first place. Many are loaded with hydrogenated oils and deadly trans fats. Add to that a huge dollop of sugar, preservatives, and artificial flavor and color, and you see how so many salad dressings qualify for the dirty dozen.

Just one tablespoon of a typical ranch dressing contains 74 calories, 70 of them coming from fat! Portion control is also an issue, with most people consuming more like 3 tablespoons per salad.

Some young women consume more than 50% of their total daily calories as salad dressing! And some dressings have more fat and calories than an entire entree!

This is a classic example of a food where simple substitutions such as those suggested in the excellent *Eat This, Not That* series really pay. For example, T.G.I. Friday's Balsamic Vinaigrette dressing has 590 sugar and fat based calories, but their Low-Fat Cilantro Lime is more reasonable 160 calories. Quizno's Honey Mustard has 500 calories and 48g fat, but their Fat-Free Balsamic Vinaigrette is just 120 calories.

The tragedy here is that salad dressing has the potential to be GOOD for you, especially by including olive oil, lemon or lime juice, pureed avocado, berry-based vinaigrettes, and other healthy fats and natural, nutrient packed ingredients.

9. Potato chips, corn chips, pretzels, and "snack" foods in general

Fat, sodium, refined carbs, weird added colors and flavors – and no redeeming neuro-nutrients, protein, or fiber. Just a whole bunch of empty calories, and all too often dangerous trans fats. I know these are another favorite "comfort food" or "self-medication", but let's quickly re-visit our goals – what we NEED is:

- stable blood sugar and stable moods

- neuro-nutrients that improve compromised bipolar brain chemistry

- nutrient dense calorie foods that make it easy to get the nourishment we need but still fight back against the weight gain effect of most bipolar drugs

- a "clean" diet that protects us from the heart disease, high blood pressure, strokes, diabetes, and other chronic physical conditions that affect people with bipolar far more than the general population.

Here we have a whole category of foods that provide NONE of these benefits, while being packed with either empty calories or active toxins. There is no short term mood boost that can make eating these "non-foods" worth it once we look at the big picture.

10. Cookies, muffins, cakes, pies ... and sorry ... donuts

Sadly, chocolate chip cookies, red velvet cake, apple pie, or whatever your preferred comfort food may be, is also another sugar/fat combo with all the pitfalls of ice cream or donuts. Baked goods have that wholesome, home-made aura, even when they come from Publix, but baked versus fried does not necessarily mean any nutritional advantages. Any sugar/fat combo is a bad food choice, and these ones have the added punch of frequently containing deadly trans fats or artificial flavors and colors that are bad for your heart, your brain chemistry, or possibly both.

Some may masquerade as "healthy" but the reality is they are dangerous traps. For example, while the Panera Pumpkin Muffin even manages to incorporate a vegetable – the truth is one of these has 530 calories and packs a whopping 47 grams of sugar.

Donuts are a lot like ice cream – a highly enjoyable, highly habit forming, culturally pervasive "All American" combo of saturated fat and refined sugar.

Typically over 50% of the calories in a donut come from saturated fat, and the actual calorie value ranges anywhere from 150 to 450 calories.

A Chocolate Frosted Cake Donut from Dunkin' Donuts contains a whopping 360 calories! Of these 50% of the calories, that is a whole 180 calories, come from fat. That is 20 grams of fat! The rest of the donut is a mere 1 gram of fiber and 40 grams of simple carbs – basically straight sugar!

11. Fast food

Confession time again. I LOVE junk food, especially McDonalds Quarter Pounders with Cheese, Sonic hot dogs, and EVERYTHING at Dairy Queen. I am such a junk food junkie that I prefer to celebrate my birthday at Dairy Queen, instead of at a fancy haute cuisine restaurant.

However, these days I know enough about how fast food impacts my bipolar disorder to save Dairy Queen just for birthdays . . . and maybe 1 or 2 other special occasions . . .

Also, just as with the ice cream business, I have several times made a living in the fast food industry, and got the money to go to college from operating a hot dog franchise back when I was 21. So I hate to criticize these products, and am not just jumping on the anti-junk food, or anti-McDonalds bandwagon. If anything I hold the rather unfashionable position that family restaurants are an important industry and make many positive contributions to society.

Unfortunately though, there is no getting away from the negative results that their food products have on customers who have bipolar or other mood disorders.

Think junk food and we are back to the usual suspects – saturated fat and refined carbohydrates. Even a relatively modest 3 ounce hot dog has 16 grams of fat, of which 7 grams are saturated. Hamburgers are almost always made from fatty meat cuts – it makes them affordable and easy to fry and grill – but it means way too much saturated fat. Add the sugar and white flour from the buns and you are on a ticket to mood swings, diabetes and clogged arteries.

How about pizza? Again, it is a classic carb and fat combo, and you are better off without it. However, some choices are better than others:

Pizza Selection	Calories	Fat	Saturated Fat
2 slices Pizza Hut Supreme Pan style	620	32	12
2 slices Pizza Hut Ham and Pineapple, Thin 'N Crispy style	360	12	6
2 slices Domino's Ultimate Deep Dish ExtravaganZZa Feast	620	34	12
2 slices Domino's Crunchy Thin Crust Pizza with Ham and Pineapple	300	16	4

These figures came from the excellent *Eat This, Not That* series, and I highly recommend the snappy little books and the website if you must have the occasional junk food fix. As you can see from the figures in the table above, your mental and physical health can benefit greatly from a few simple but informed substitutions.

12. Alcohol

A relationship between mood disorders and alcohol has been observed for over 2,000 years, dating back to the writings of Plato, who believed that abusing alcohol could induce episodes of mania. Individuals with bipolar disorder have a particularly high risk of developing a drinking problem. Some studies put the risk at around 49%, compared to only 13% for the general population. We know from the research that some people drink when they are manic in order to prolong and intensify feelings of elation, whereas others drink when depressed as a form of self-medication in order to numb the pain. Some do both.

Research into the effects of drinking on people with manic-depressive illness show the following risks when alcohol and bipolar mix:

- disturbed sleep
- increased impulsivity
- increased aggression
- more mixed states
- more rapid cycling

- higher suicide risks (a drunk person is more likely to successfully complete a suicide attempt than to fumble it)
- more unemployment
- more divorce
- more legal problems
- greater likelihood of mild drinking escalating into alcoholism.

What type of alcohol you consume may make a difference. Research shows that beer in moderation (2-3 a week) does not have the same level of risk as 2-3 weekly drinks of spirits.

However, overall there are so many reasons for a person with bipolar disorder to avoid all forms of alcohol that it is overwhelming. Alcohol impairs judgment and does away with inhibitions, compounding two of bipolar disorder's most destructive characteristics.

If you are depressed, alcohol will make you more depressed, and the effect of this compounds over time. Up to 70% of alcoholics suffer from chronic depression. Alcohol depletes omega-3s and also lowers your brain's levels of tryptophan and disrupts serotonin production.

If you are manic, alcohol is literally fuel to the fire and encourages more dangerous and destructive behaviors, especially when it comes to money, sex, aggression, and suicide.

If you are on medication (and medication is after all, the most effective and common treatment for bipolar), alcohol can compound side effects such as sleepiness, foggy thinking or sexual dysfunction.

Combined with sedatives like Valium or Klonopin it can cause respiratory failure (you quit breathing and die). Lithium, the most established mood stabilizer for bipolar disorder, must be maintained at precise levels in the blood. Alcohol interferes with this and creates serious risks of toxicity and kidney damage, as well as compromising the medicine's effectiveness.

Alcohol also dehydrates the body and this increases fatigue, irritability and the inability to concentrate.

It also disrupts sleep – a critical issue in manic depression. Our illness is associated with extra sensitive body clocks and the need to maintain healthy and stable circadian rhythms and get adequate sleep.

A whole book could be written about why alcohol is potential poison for manic depressives. Please minimize your drinking or abstain completely. I have always loved to drink, but after cutting back dramatically I find I no longer want or enjoy liquor, and now genuinely enjoy life more without it.

Chapter 4: Is Your Medication Making You Fat?

One of the most common barriers to recovery is non-compliance with taking medication. In fact, in working with people with manic-depressive illness, I have reached the point where every day now I hear the same story from either someone under treatment or their spouse – "Everything was fine until I/he/she stopped taking the meds".

Now I do not for one moment believe that people with bipolar disorder are stupid, and that they do not understand the relationship between taking meds and staying well. In fact, it is well accepted that folks with bipolar disorder tend to be, if anything, smarter than the average bear.

My belief is that for the most part, these wonderful people are not making naïve, capricious or irresponsible decisions. I suspect that for many of us, we go off our meds because we have performed our own personal cost/benefit analysis and decided that because we are managing better we can afford to risk an episode in exchange for a period of relief from medication side effects.

And as vain or shallow as it may sound to the uninitiated, the number one side effect that many of us hate the most is weight gain.

Nearly every effective medication for bipolar disorder has weight gain as a side effect. However, it is important to remember that not everyone taking a particular drug will experience side effects. NEVER let the fear of a particular side effect prevent you from trying a medication that your doctor (ideally an experienced psychiatrist with specific expertise in bipolar disorder) believes could be helpful for you.

The fact is that we all respond differently to the various mood stabilizers and other medications, and some folks will never gain an ounce. However, weight gain is extremely common, and if you are unhappy with your current weight, it may be relevant for you to ask "Is my medication making me fat?"

If the weight gain began at the same time as you started taking the meds, the answer is probably yes.

However, in the US and other developed countries, we are in the middle of an obesity epidemic. The issues around weight and bipolar disorder are complex and interrelated. Understanding what is going on in relation to your own weight gain, and turning things around, is going to take concentration and dedicated effort.

Did you start to gain weight before commencing medications? There is no shame in it if you did. In fact, it puts you in the majority. 70% of American men and over 60% of women are overweight, and approximately one third of the US population is obese – and it just gets worse every year.

Some research has been done on whether people with bipolar disorder start off being heavier than the general population, even before diagnosis and treatment, but the results have been mixed. What we do know is that after being diagnosed and treated, weight management is a huge issue for the bipolar population, with 35% of people with bipolar disorder being obese! This is the highest percentage of any psychiatric illness!

It is also important to consider the high percentage of people with bipolar disorder who also have reactive hyperglycemia, together with heightened risk factors for carb and fat fueled diseases such as heart disease, stroke and diabetes.

Hence the emphasis in *The Bipolar Diet* on a high protein diet, and a focus on "good" carbs and "healthy" fats. The extra weight gain caused by medication can push you over the edge. Cutting way back on the sugar, white bread, and saturated fat will not just improve your moods – it may save your life. Fight back with smart food choices, an enjoyable exercise plan you can stick with, and a realistic assessment of what your weight should be. All of this will be covered as you progress through this book ☺

I get more questions about meds and weight gain than anything else, and I KNOW that many people quit taking their medication because they find the weight gain to be so extremely demoralizing. Much as I sympathize with this (and believe me – I do – after gaining over 40 pounds I did it myself) it is NOT the answer. Instead, learn about the weight gain/loss implications of the various meds that are used to treat bipolar disorder, and the strategies you can use to maintain your weight at a healthy level where you can feel good about yourself.

Which meds are most likely to cause weight gain?

Brand Name(s)	Generic	Heavy Gain	Significant Gain	Weight Neutral
Clozapine, Clozaril, Clopine	Clozapine	X		
Zyprexa, Zyprexa Zydis, Zalasta, Zolafren, Olzapin	Olanzapine	X		

Brand Name(s)	Generic	Heavy Gain	Significant Gain	Weight Neutral
Seroquel, Ketipinor	Quetiapine		X	
Risperdal, Ridal, Sizodon, Riscalin, Rispolept, Rispen	Risperidone		X	
Eskalith, Eskalith-Cr, Lithane	Lithium		X	
Depakote, Epival, Encorate Chrono, Divalpro	Valproate		X	
Neurontin	Gabapentin		X	
Prozac, Lexapro, Zoloft, and so on.	SSRI antidepressants		X	
Geodon, Zeldox	Ziprasidone			X
Abilify, Abilify Discmelt	Aripiprazole			X
Tegretol, Biston, Carbatrol, Epitol, Carbamaze, Degranol	Carbamazepine			X
Lamictal, Lamictin, Lamogine	Lamotrigine			X

Talking to your doctor

Don't be afraid to discuss this with the medical professional who prescribes your drugs. If you have bipolar disorder there are a range of medication options available - it is perfectly ok for you to ask for one that has fewer side effects and that will not undermine your overall health!

For instance, Zyprexa, a drug manufactured by Eli-Lilly, has, in the last few years, been the target of multiple lawsuits across the country. In particular, it is alleged that taking Zyprexa can cause excessive weight gain and even diabetes. If your doctor recommends Zyprexa to treat your bipolar disorder, talk to him about the risks of these potential side effects and ask about the possibility of a safer alternative.

Ask your doctor politely but firmly about trying Lamictal or Abilify. Sometimes side effects such as panic attacks or the notorious "Lamictal rash" will rule these alternative meds out, but usually they are safe to try.

Some doctors offer a cocktail of meds to help counteract the weight gain. For example Wellbutrin, especially if you are on an anti-convulsant, or Topomax. (I have tried both. Wellbutrin was very good for me, but Topomax made me a zombie who couldn't speak in sentences and mixed up words.)

What is important is that your doctor be proactive in helping you find medication that stabilizes moods without destroying your overall health through substantial weight gain.

Fending off the fat

Exercise! Exercise! Exercise! Also, you will need to use a combination of calorie counting and portion control to avoid overeating. As a person with bipolar disorder, you have increased risk factors for heart disease, diabetes and stroke, so sensible eating is necessary for more than just weight control. It is possible that you may need to change your eating patterns, especially if you have previously consumed lots of carbs or junk food. Don't worry. The improvement in your moods, physical health, appearance, and self-respect will make the changes more than worth it. And the guidelines explained to you here in *The Bipolar Diet* will make it easy ☺

Finding the balance

Everyone has a different body weight at which they are comfortable. Many of us accept a little weight gain as we get older and realize that the uber-thin models on the magazine covers are not realistic or attractive. Don't get too hung-up on gaining a few pounds, especially if the alternative is crippling bouts of depression and/or mania that can destroy relationships, careers, finances, and families.

NEVER go off your meds simply to lose weight, especially if you have a history of reckless behavior or self-harm.

NEVER take diet pills. They are dangerous anyway, but for a person with bipolar disorder you are risking mania, cardiovascular damage – even death.

But do get a grip. For me, a gain of 10-20 pounds is ok. I can live with it. A gain of 50 or 70 pounds is a different story!

Monitor other factors such as cholesterol, iron, thyroid hormone, blood fats, blood pressure, insulin – not just your weight.

Your focus needs to be on holistic wellness. That means a healthy mind AND a healthy body. If your meds stabilize your mood, your physical health indicators remain positive (low cholesterol, low blood pressure etc), but you have gained 10 pounds, then maybe you need to reframe your ideas about body image. However, regardless of whether you have gained 50 lbs or 5 lbs, if you show the danger signs of mounting risk of heart attack, stroke or diabetes, then obviously things have to change!

Chapter 5: The Bipolar Thyroid Connection

According to Drs Goodwin and Jamison in *Manic-Depressive Illness: Bipolar Disorders and Recurrent Depression:* "Thyroid dysfunction associated with bipolar disorder is a significant problem".

What is the bipolar/thyroid connection?

The thyroid is a large, butterfly shaped gland in the neck. A normally functioning thyroid uses iodine and the amino acid tyrosine to produce exactly the right amounts of the important thyroid hormones thyroxine (T4) and triiodothyronine (T3). Through these thyroid hormones, the thyroid controls many important bodily functions, including:

- regulating metabolism (how quickly the body burns energy)
- production of proteins
- sensitivity to proteins.

The thyroid hormones produced by the thyroid gland are responsible for how every cell in your body converts oxygen and calories to energy. However, sometimes the thyroid malfunctions and does not produce the very precise and balanced amounts of T3 and T4 needed for optimal health. There are two ways things can get out of whack:

1. Underactive thyroid = too little thyroid hormone, which results in hypothyroidism.

2. Overactive thyroid = too much thyroid hormone, which results in hyperthyroidism.

People who have a thyroid gland that is not functioning properly are more likely to have bipolar disorder, panic disorder, OCD, major depression, and/or a whole range of other mood disorders than the population in general.

Research such as the STEP-BD clinical study has shown that the connection between thyroid problems and bipolar disorder is far more common amongst women than men. Also, Bipolar II or "soft bipolar" is more strongly connected to thyroid disorders than Bipolar I. There is also a link between rapid cycling and hypothyroidism. (Hypothyroidism, which means an under-active thyroid is the most frequent manifestation of thyroid dysfunction.)

ALL people suffering from bipolar disorder should also be carefully screened by their doctor(s) for the other mental and physical health complications that commonly occur along with bipolar, for example substance abuse, anxiety disorders, heart disease, diabetes and so forth. However, based on the information above, it is particularly important that ALL WOMEN WITH BIPOLAR II ALWAYS BE CHECKED FOR AN UNDER-ACTIVE THYROID.

Common thyroid dysfunction symptoms

Psychiatric Symptoms of Hypothyroidism	Psychiatric Symptoms of Hyperthyroidism
- Depression	- Anxiety
- Cognitive dysfunction	- Restlessness
- Irritability	- Exaggerated emotional responses, such as laughing or crying, that is uncontrollable out of proportion.
- Memory loss	- Feelings of unhappiness and dissatisfaction

Physical Symptoms of Hypothyroidism	Physical Symptoms of Hyperthyroidism
- Fatigue	- Heart palpitations or rapid heart beat
- Weight gain	- Insomnia
- Dry skin	- Breathlessness
- Intolerance to cold	- Weight loss
- Coarse dry hair	- Increased bowel movements
- Weakness and/or muscle aches	- Light or absent menstrual periods
- Loss of libido	- Trembling hands
- Abnormal menstrual cycles	- Warm moist skin
- Constipation	- Staring gaze

Note that in the table above, I have included symptoms of over active thyroid (hyperthyroidism) for the sake of completeness. However, there is little compelling evidence of a strong link between hyperthyroidism and bipolar disorder – it is the link between bipolar and hypothyroidism that is supported by consistent and plentiful data. The rest of this chapter will only discuss the under active thyroid because that is what is most relevant to us.

What is an "under-active" thyroid?

This is where things get extremely interesting for people with bipolar disorder, but also a tad confusing. The problem is that the whole notion of what is an adequate, "normal" level of thyroid hormone is increasingly debated and controversial.

Usually when you have blood work done, your doctor will base treatment decisions on what the lab where your blood was tested has flagged as "out of range" versus "normal" in their report. Currently, the majority of US labs report the "normal" reference range for the

Thyroid Stimulating Hormone (TSH) as being between 0.5 – 5.0.

However, as long ago as January 2003, the American Association of Clinical Endocrinologists, started advising doctors that a more accurate range would be a range of TSH level from 0.3 - 3.0. This means that based on the latest medical evidence, millions of Americans have low thyroid function in the TSH range of 3.0 – 5.0 but are not getting identified in the lab reports relied on by their family doctor. Using the updated range would put 20% of the population as hypothyroid, as opposed to just 5% as measured now. Some experts even believe the correct range should be even narrower, at 0.4 - 2.5. (You can read a simple description of the research on About.com's Thyroid Testing webpage.)

THIS MEANS YOU COULD BE HYPOTHYROID, DESPITE WHAT A BLOOD TEST SAYS.

On top of the confusion around testing ranges, studies have shown that many people with bipolar disorder, particularly those who are in depressive episodes, have "subclinical" low levels of thyroid hormone – they do not meet the "official" diagnosis of hypothyroid with a TSH of over 5.0, but their TSH is still at the low end of the scale.

It boils down to this: thyroid malfunction is a very important complication in bipolar disorder, but is commonly overlooked. It is imperative that you have your thyroid function tested immediately if you have been diagnosed with bipolar disorder. If your thyroid function level is low but "normal" (that is, if your TSH is in the range of 2.5 – 5.0), or definitely low by even the out-dated standard (TSH over 5.0), then starting thyroid supplementation immediately is likely to be highly beneficial.

Also please understand: in modern developed nations there is so much iodine in our diet that thyroid malfunction is not related to malnutrition, and you cannot boost your thyroid back to normal through natural supplements based on vitamins or minerals. If you are low on thyroid, you will need to take thyroid hormone supplements to correct the problem. Testing your thyroid function and augmenting thyroid hormones where necessary should be the first step in treatment of bipolar depression, right alongside prescribing a mood stabilizer.

An excellent book for the lay reader is *Thyroid Power* by Richard Shames, M.D. and Karilee Shames, R.N., PH.D. It describes how fatigue, weight gain, depression, high cholesterol, low sex drive, and a host of other difficulties are often due to low thyroid. It also explains how to talk to your doctor about misconceptions about hypothyroidism, and what is really "normal".

Chapter 6:
Supplements for Bipolar?

Every day I get messages on the Bipolar-Lives website, asking advice about treating bipolar disorder with vitamins and nutritional supplements instead of medication.

It seems many people prefer the idea of taking something "natural". Also, as many of us have discovered through years of unpleasant trial and error, the side effects of bipolar meds are no fun, and it is easy to understand why some people seek to avoid taking these drugs.

In my experience, medication is life-saving and usually a necessity. Some very mild cases of Bipolar II (and I mean VERY MILD – the softest of soft bipolar) may be effectively treated through diet and lifestyle alone, but only an experienced clinician could advise you on that. Following *The Bipolar Diet* is intended to promote stable moods, protect against unwanted medication side effects such as weight gain, and promote greater physical and mental health overall – it is not a substitute for professional care and medication.

Ironically, lithium IS a natural cure. It is a naturally occurring mineral salt and has more in common with nutritional supplements than with artificial pharmaceuticals. (You can read more about lithium here.)

The natural health industry is a multi-billion dollar corporate monster in just the same way as Big-Pharma is. Also, because products are not FDA approved, many misleading claims abound, and it is easy to waste time and money on products that are long on hype and short on science.

Don't get me wrong – I am NOT opposed to natural approaches – the whole premise of this book is that people suffering from manic-depressive illness can dramatically improve their mental AND physical health through wise nutritional approaches and supplementing with PROVEN natural supplements. I know because I have done it. I am living proof! However, I would be ashamed to admit how much money I have wasted over the years on supplements that did no good, or that actually made my episodes worse. Today I am very careful to make sure there is reliable research on ANY vitamin, herb, or other supplement I put in my body.

My friend Tom Venuto has summarized some of these issues brilliantly in his wonderful e-book *Burn the Fat, Feed the Muscle:*

> *"You should always be skeptical about any drug-like claims that are made for over-the-counter supplements. Whenever a supplement company releases a new product, The Food & Drug Administration (FDA) has their eyes on it with a magnifying glass. So does the pharmaceutical industry. If any "natural" or "herbal" product really had a major effect on the body, the FDA would swoop down on it like a hawk and investigate immediately. If it panned out and really did have drug-like effects, it would be pulled off the shelves in a heartbeat! . . . Also keep in mind that the powerful multi-billion dollar pharmaceutical industry would LOVE to find a product being sold over the counter that really had drug-like effects, and lobby*

to have it classified as a drug. Why? So they could quadruple the price and sell it by prescription only (with some fancy new drug-like name, of course)."

(If you are not familiar with Tom's work, you should be. His *Burn the Fat, Feed the Muscle* is one of the best-selling e-books of all time. In fact, it has been at the top of the fat-loss bestsellers for 7 years in a row! My book, *The Bipolar Diet,* is great for balancing moods and maintaining a healthy weight, but if you want to get seriously ripped and have the body of professional fitness model, check out Tom's tips on food, exercise – and supplements ☺)

The real tragedy is that some supplements do show great promise for treating depression and even mania, but because they cannot be patented and turned into zillion-dollar cash cows, usually there is just not enough interest to conduct enough rigorous scientific studies to prove their effectiveness.

Based on the evidence, here are some suggestions of what to try, and what to avoid:

5-HTP

5-HTP (5-hydroxytryptophan) is a naturally occurring amino acid. It is considered to have potential as a mood supporter because it is a precursor to the neurotransmitter serotonin and is also involved in metabolizing tryptophan. In the US it has been heavily marketed as an antidepressant, appetite suppressant, and sleep aid. However, according to a 2001 overview of the research, there is insufficient high quality research to prove that 5-HTP is really effective.

According to Consumer Reports Health.org, 5-HTP has documented side effects including severe gastrointestinal symptoms and pain and inflammation of the muscles, joints, and skin.

Verdict: No proven effectiveness for bipolar disorder or any other health benefits. Don't bother.

Choline

Choline is a water-soluble essential nutrient, usually grouped within the Vitamin B complex. It is a natural amine and has potential for the treatment of bipolar disorder because it helps make up the neurotransmitter acetylcholine. Acetylcholine affects memory, intelligence and mood. Acetylcholine levels on the brain can be increased through choline supplementation. One trial showed that 204 grams a day of choline per day was effective in reducing both manic and depressive symptoms. This is a promising finding but it was only a preliminary trial. No properly controlled trials have yet investigated the effects of choline in treating people with bipolar disorder. Until there are proper double-blind studies performed it is impossible to render a verdict.

Try it if you are not getting results from meds or other supplements, otherwise wait for more information.

Folic acid

Folic acid is also known as folate. It is part of the family of B vitamins, and is an important building block for DNA, and essential to cell replication and growth. Many people are deficient in folic acid, although there are many rich dietary sources such as leafy green vegetables and meat. Some breakfast cereals are fortified with folic acid.

Deficiencies are especially common amongst alcoholics and heavy drinkers, women taking birth control pills, pregnant women, the elderly (especially African-Americans), and people taking anticonvulsant medication. Folic acid deficiency has been found among people with depression and has been linked to poor response to antidepressant treatment. One study has also linked low folic acid levels to mania. Some evidence has suggested a tendency to deficiency amongst people with bipolar disorder, but other studies did not replicate this.

It does seem clear that taking folic acid, especially in combination with B12, is helpful for depression and possibly mania, although more research is needed to clarify the value of folic acid for treating mania and mood swings, as opposed to depression.

Folic acid supplementation can mask vitamin B12 deficiency, so make sure you are getting plenty of both.

Doses of 400 – 800 mcg of folic acid daily are suggested.

For more information and details on specific clinical studies, see the Bipolar Lives website page on the Benefits of Folic Acid.

GABA

GABA (gamma-aminobutyric acid) is an amino acid which is also classified as a neurotransmitter. It is believed to have a calming and relaxing effect as it is an inhibitory neurotransmitter which balances the excitation of the brain with inhibition. Decreased levels of GABA have been found in the brain, cerebrospinal fluid, and plasma of people with bipolar disorder. However, due to side effects and difficulties with GABA crossing the blood brain barrier, plus a lack of any clinical studies, the known link between bipolar disorder and GABA deficiency does not translate into the use of GABA as a supplement that will safely and effectively treat bipolar disorder.

Cover your bases by eating GABA rich foods such as through the high protein Bipolar Diet, but don't bother spending money on GABA supplements to treat your bipolar as there is no compelling evidence that they can help you.

Inositol

Regular readers of my Bipolar Lives website will know I was an early advocate for supplementing with high doses of inositol. However, as I have studied more of the research it seems the results of the clinical studies are not just inconclusive but downright contradictory! At this stage I regard inositol with more caution and do not believe the evidence is strong enough to be certain that the benefits of taking inositol outweigh possible risks.

If you take it and it works for you great. If you have not tried inositol, watch this space and I will update when the evidence becomes clearer.

Magnesium

Magnesium is a mineral and is an essential component of a healthy diet. However, most of us run the risk of magnesium deficiency, with only 32% of Americans getting their recommended daily allowance (RDA). Nuts and leafy green vegetables are good sources of magnesium. Also, magnesium is usually included in any common multi-vitamin and mineral supplement. You can get enough magnesium from taking one of these and you don't need to spend any extra money on additional magnesium supplementation. It can be helpful for many health problems, including headaches, PMS, high cholesterol, the metabolic syndrome that signals the approach of diabetes, and also may decrease the risk of stroke. Magnesium metabolism is very important to insulin sensitivity and blood pressure regulation, and magnesium deficiency is common in individuals with diabetes. The observed associations between magnesium metabolism, diabetes, and high blood pressure increase the likelihood that magnesium metabolism may influence cardiovascular disease. It is therefore an important supplement for people with bipolar disorder as they have an increased risk of diabetes, heart disease and stroke. However, there is no evidence to show that magnesium is useful for mood stabilization.

Eat nuts and green vegetables and take your daily multi-vitamin and mineral supplement with up to 350 mgs of magnesium per day. Magnesium matters!

Multivitamin and mineral supplements

Multivitamin and mineral supplements are a great insurance policy that ensure your basic needs are being met. In some cases they can supply high enough doses of the vitamins and minerals known to be useful in treating bipolar disorder that no extra supplementation is necessary.

In 2002, the *Journal of the American Medical Association* stated that "*it appears prudent for all adults to take vitamin supplements.*" A 1998 issue of the *New England Journal of Medicine* featured an editorial entitled "*Eat Right and Take a Multivitamin*" that was based on studies that showed health benefits resulting from the consumption of nutritional supplements.

Look for a supplement that includes:

- Folic acid
- Magnesium
- Vitamin B12
- Vitamin C
- Zinc.

You will needs to take your fish oil (omega-3) separately. If you wish to try the amino acids taurine and tyrosine these will probably also need to be taken separately. (See below.)

Omega-3 (fish oil)

Fish oils can be obtained from eating fish or by taking supplements. Fish oil benefits include:

- Protection from bipolar relapse.
- Relief from unipolar and bipolar depression.
- Protection from heart disease and stroke.
- Lowers the risk of type 1 diabetes.

It would be reasonable to ask why there is so little attention paid to effective nutritional supplements such as fish oil.

According to Goodwin's and Jamison's *"Manic-Depressive Illness: Bipolar Disorders and Recurrent Depression"* (2nd ed), 2007, the most authoritative medical text on bipolar: *"Because nutritional supplements cannot be patented, there is no large industrial base of support for research on these compounds. . . clinical research thus far, while not definitive, has yielded some encouraging results . . . about the addition of omega-3 fatty acids [fish oil]."*

Basically any drug getting these sorts of results for bipolar depression would be heavily funded with lots of studies and applications to the FDA.

Fortunately however, there are enough responsible clinicians like Goodwin and Jamison that the medical establishment has not completely overlooked healthy alternatives such as fish oil, and good research does exist.

Interest in fish oil benefits for bipolar was initially sparked by studies that found lower rates of major depression and suicidal thinking in countries where people naturally consumed large amounts of fish oil as part of their regular diets. Clinicians became interested in conducting research into fish oil benefits for bipolar people because of these observations that there seemed to be a link between high levels of fish oil consumption and low rates of bipolar and depression.

There have been several controlled studies showing fish oil benefits as an add-on to other medication. This means that it is a very good idea to take fish oil in addition to your regular medication.

As yet, there is not enough research to prove fish oil alone can effectively treat bipolar disorder. The clinical evidence and the benefits shown in these studies are discussed in more detail on the Bipolar Lives website – see Fish Oil Benefits at http://www.bipolar-lives.com/fish-oil-benefits.html.

Try a dose of 1 gram a day. Go up to 2 after a month if you do not feel any benefits.

SAMe

SAMe (S-Adenosylmethionine) is a form of the amino acid methionine, and is a naturally occurring chemical that is found throughout the human body. According to the Mayo Clinic: *"SAMe has been studied for use in depression for many decades, however, currently available trials are inconclusive."* However, it has been used as a prescription antidepressant in Europe for a decade, and other experts such as Drs Goodwin and Jamison cite research studies that do show SAMe to be an effective antidepressant. The problem with SAMe is that in some trials it has been shown to induce mania, and even those who acknowledge SAMe's antidepressant qualities advise it should be avoided by people with bipolar disorder. Don't risk it.

St. John's Wort

St. John's Wort is an herb, also known as hypericum perforatum. It is probably effective for treating mild depression, but the research does not establish effectiveness for serious depression. Like SAMe, St. John's Wort has been shown to induce mania. Also, it can interact with many other medications and should not be used without medical supervision.

Although the common wisdom is that this is a safe and natural antidepressant, experts such as the Mayo Clinic, Consumer Reports Health.org, and Drs Goodwin and Jamison in their textbook *Manic-Depressive Illness,* all advise that people with bipolar disorder should NOT take St John's Wort. Avoid!

Taurine

Taurine is a non-essential amino acid. It occurs mainly in foods such as meat and fish, and this is one of the many reasons why *The Bipolar Diet* emphasizes eating plenty of lean protein. Many factors can lead to taurine deficiency, for example stress and low vitamin B6. Taurine shows up frequently in trendy energy drinks, but it has not been shown to have any energy-giving properties. Rather, it is an anti-anxiety agent, and also has antioxidant properties, and supports brain and heart functioning. It may be of value to people with bipolar disorder in addressing both mental and physical health issues. It assists cardiovascular function, cholesterol elimination, and reduces hyper tension. However, of most interest is the way taurine can stabilize nerve cell membranes, which prevents the erratic firing of nerve cells. Like many bipolar medications, taurine is an anti-convulsant and mild sedative. It has been shown to help treat epilepsy and other excitable brain states. It has been suggested to have good potential in treating bipolar disorder but must be taken in modest doses as too much taurine can cause depression and short term memory loss. The Mayo Clinic states that: *"Up to 3,000 milligrams of supplemental taurine a day is considered safe. Any excess taurine is simply excreted by the kidneys. Moderation is important, however. Little is known about the effects of heavy or long-term taurine use."* A sensible dose to try would be 1,000 mg daily.

Tyrosine

Tyrosine is another non-essential amino acid. It is found in high protein foods such as chicken, turkey, fish, almonds, and also in avocados. There are several reasons for supplementing with tyrosine. It provides important metabolic support and aids fat loss. Also, it is a precursor to the 3 important "feel good" neurotransmitters - dopamine, norepinephrine and epinephrine. These regulate and elevate mood and are common targets of bipolar medications. Tyrosine is believed to also support the adrenal and thyroid glands, and can reduce anxiety and depression. Interestingly, the studies show it to be effective in people who are stressed, rather than "normal". The suggested dose is 500-1500 mg per day, split into 3 separate doses. DO NOT TAKE TYROSINE IF YOU ARE ALSO TAKING AN MAO inhibitor. (BTW: I started learning about both taurine and tyrosine on the About.com: Bipolar Disorder: Nutrition pages. This is a great resource for anyone interested in the role of nutrition in treating bipolar disorder.)

Vitamin B12

Vitamin B12 is an essential water-soluble vitamin that is commonly found in a variety of foods such as fish, shellfish, meat, and dairy products. According to the Mayo Clinic: *"A day's supply of vitamin B12 can be obtained by eating 1 chicken breast plus 1 hard-boiled egg plus 1 cup plain low-fat yogurt, or 1 cup milk plus 1 cup raisin bran."* B12 is essential for the normal functioning of the human brain and nervous system. Although B12 deficiency is rare, it is extremely serious. Vitamin B12 deficiency, even at levels only slightly lower than normal, can cause fatigue, depression, and poor memory. B12 deficiency can also cause symptoms of mania and psychosis. However, supplementation of 2-3 mcg per day of B12 through a multi-vitamin and mineral supplement should be enough to protect you.

One expert has published research suggesting 1 mg daily for treating depression.

Get your B12 levels tested if you are elderly, vegetarian, vegan, or simply worried about B12 deficiency. Although the potential is high for a B12 deficiency to produce bipolar symptoms, there is no published research to show B12 supplementation assists people with bipolar disorder. My approach is to take it in safe amounts as it is useful for depression and general brain function.

Vitamin C

Vitamin C deficiency has been observed in people with bipolar disorder, but there is no compelling evidence to suggest vitamin C can help to stabilize moods. However, there are other reasons for making sure you have adequate vitamin C. It helps with iron absorption and many people with bipolar are also anemic. It also may help reduce blood pressure and improve circulation. Severe lack of vitamin C leads to the disease scurvy. Be aware that vitamin C can be a double-edged sword and that talk of it preventing heart disease and lowering cholesterol is not supported by the research. You should NOT take vitamin C in doses greater than those found in basic multivitamins if you have had a heart attack, a heart procedure, or you have diabetes. You definitely need your RDA of vitamin C but there is no special reason for a person with bipolar disorder to take elevated doses.

(Some evidence suggests that bipolar people have elevated levels of a substance called vanadium, and that taking vitamin C reduces vanadium to normal and alleviates bipolar symptoms but this is very speculative and does not support heavy vitamin C supplementation until more and better research on the topic proves the connection.)

This is another one that you can address through your daily multi so don't waste money or increase risk of complications from heart disease or diabetes.

Zinc

Zinc is an essential mineral which plays an important role in the human diet. Some of the best dietary sources are red meats such as beef and lamb. Although many people in developing countries are deficient in zinc, in the US and other developed nations the average dietary intake of zinc is usually sufficient. However, zinc is almost always included in popular vitamin and mineral supplements, despite the fact that most of us get enough as part of our regular diet. There is no evidence that zinc is useful for bipolar disorder, although it MAY be helpful for depression associated with eating disorders. It is true that we all need zinc as part of our daily diet, and zinc is associated with a range of physical health benefits. However, most people get enough zinc from their regular food. If not, taking a typical multi-vitamin/mineral complex will cover your bases. Don't spend money on extra zinc.

Chapter 7:
Winning Strategies:
Portions & Planning

Portion control and meal planning are crucial in any diet that leads to improved overall health and weight management – and in giving you a healthy and enjoyable eating plan you can stick with.

The Bipolar Diet is effective because you can happily follow it for the rest of your life. Overly restrictive, "quick-fix" diets tend to fail because they are simply too hard to stick with, make life a misery, and may actually contribute to mood swings. Instead, I suggest you use tricks like portion control, smart substitutions, and occasional indulgences to ensure *The Bipolar Diet* becomes a healthy way of life that delivers long-term, lasting benefits.

This doesn't mean you can change scientific reality - If you eat 100 more food calories a day than you burn, you'll gain nearly 1 pound in a month. That's 10 -11 pounds in a year. The bottom line is that to lose weight, it's important to reduce calories and increase physical activity. However, you must do it the smart way. A very restrictive diet can slow down your metabolism because your body goes into "starvation mode" and does everything it can to conserve body weight. The most effective approach is to have a small calorie deficit so that your metabolism stays active and burns fat. (See *Chapter 8: Meal Plans* for more about the "starvation response".)

Portion control is something you have to do for yourself, especially if you live in a country like the US where the trend is to "super-size" everything. Think about it . . . fast food has been around for a long time, but it is only in the last 20 years that obesity has become an epidemic. Why? The answer is the current emphasis on huge, out of control portions.

When McDonald's first opened, a soda was 7 ounces. Today, the child size is 12 ounces, a small is 16 ounces, and the large 32 ounces.

This is why YOU have to take charge of portion control for yourself:

Based on Portions Today Compared to 20 Years Ago			
Source of Information: The National Heart, Lung, and Blood Institute (NHLBI)			
Food Item	Calories 20 Years Ago	Calories Today	Increased Calories
Cheeseburger	333	590	257
French Fries	210	610	400
Soda	85	250	165
Spaghetti and meatballs	500	1,025	525
Turkey sandwich	320	820	500
Bagel	140	350	210
Pizza	500	850	350
Caesar salad	390	790	400
Cheesecake	260	640	380
Cookie	55	275	220

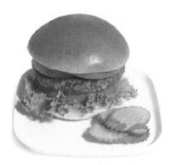
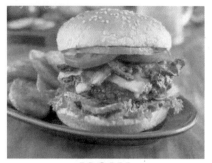

THEN   NOW

Portion Control: The basics

When you do drive up to that fast-food restaurant, don't just think about the food you will eat - think about the size or portion of the food you'll consume. Consider a child sized meal or order a salad with your burger instead of high-fat fries. A small hamburger actually goes a long way toward satisfying hunger. This was a lesson I learned from visiting a McDonald's in Thailand. The portion size was about a third of what you get in the United States – at first it seems like a rip off, but it really is enough to satisfy cravings and provide your body with sufficient fuel.

Mega-size, super-size, and extra-large portions lead to unnecessary over-eating and spikes and crashes in your blood sugar – and mood swings!

Portion control becomes second nature with practice, but to begin with you need to retrain yourself about what a healthy portion looks like, and be mindful and disciplined. You'll look, feel, and act better when you're more in control of the decisions you make about what you eat and when you eat. Important questions to ask are things like: "does it make sense for me to have a doughnut just because I'm stressed?" Or, "do I really need to eat six chocolate chip cookies to be satisfied?"

A great strategy is to downsize your dishes. A study conducted among 85 food experts revealed that when using large bowls, the experts served 31 percent more ice cream than they did when they used smaller bowls.

Using dishes that help you with portion control is a great way to manage the amount of food you eat: At home we use lovely crystal salad plates for our main meals and automatically serve and eat less – visual cues are what portion control is all about, so study the comparisons and the pictures in the next section carefully.

Visual cues for portion sizes

Grain Products	What One Serving Looks Like
1 cup of cereal flakes	The size of a fist
1 pancake	A compact disc
½ cup of cooked rice, pasta, or potato	½ of a baseball
1 slice of bread	A cassette tape

Fruits and Veggies	What One Serving Looks Like
1 cup of salad greens	A baseball
1 medium fruit	A baseball
½ cup of raisins	A large egg

Dairy and Cheese	What One Serving Looks Like
1 ½ oz. cheese	4 stacked dice
½ cup of ice cream	½ baseball
1 cup serving of milk, yogurt, or fresh greens	The size of a fist

Meats and Alternatives	What One Serving Looks Like
3 oz. meat, fish, and poultry	Deck of cards
3 oz. grilled/baked fish	Checkbook

2 Tbsp. peanut butter	Ping pong ball
Fats	**What One Serving Looks Like**
1 teaspoon of oil	The size of your thumb tip

Don't worry - visualizing portions soon becomes second-nature. For some people, it is easier to visualize portion sizes when compared to everyday items. In addition to the above table, another technique for visualizing proper portions is to see pictures of items that are basically the equivalent size of a portion. See the pictures below:

Thickness of a sandwich with ham or turkey, lettuce, and tomato should be about the size of a ballpoint pen.

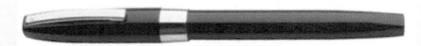

A slice of bread should be about the size of a cassette tape.

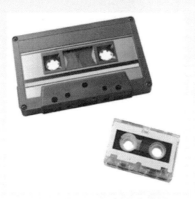

½ Cup of Almonds is about the size of a large egg

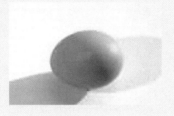

Meal Planning: How much should you eat?

Portion control is a great way to prevent unconscious overeating. As my grandmother would say, it can help you "stop digging your grave with your teeth".

As explained above, portion control allows you to indulge in "cheat" foods such as those listed in the "Dirty Dozen" in a controlled way that will minimize the negative impact on mental and physical health. However, if you experienced serious weight gain, which happens to many people taking bipolar medications, then shedding fat will require counting calories – at least in the beginning.

Regardless of whether your goal is to gain weight, lose weight, or maintain your existing weight, the information that follows is the most precise guide you will find to calculating a healthy body weight and the precise number of calories to achieve/maintain it.

WARNING: This does get a little detailed and technical, but once you master the basics it is easy to make accurate calculations, and to update your calorie requirements to allow for changes in your weight or level of physical activity. We will be looking at how to calculate the three most important numbers you need to be aware of:

1. Your body fat percentage
2. Your percentage of muscle
3. Calories required to maintain existing body weight.

Once you know these 3 critical variables, you can easily figure out how to:

1. Maintain your current weight
2. Lose body fat while retaining muscle
3. Gain weight, with an emphasis on gaining healthy lean muscle instead of dangerous fat.

How much should I weigh?

The Bipolar Diet has 3 goals:

1. Minimizing mood swings through stabilizing blood sugar and insulin response
2. Protecting against heart disease, stroke, diabetes and other physical diseases that particularly "target" people with bipolar disorder
3. Controlling weight, especially for the many people that have gained weight due to their bipolar medications.

Healthy weight is actually related to all 3 of these goals – not just weight loss.

However, there are many confusing messages around what a healthy weight really is – everything from out-dated height and weight tables from the insurance companies, to media images of impossibly slender models, complicated formulas like the Body Mass Index (BMI), and even well-meaning but unhelpful shrinks who like to say things to us like "Would you rather be crazy or fat?"

The premise of *The Bipolar Diet* is that the best way to maintain a healthy weight for you as an individual is to target a healthy weight RANGE based on BODY COMPOSITION. Body composition is the breakdown between your body's muscle, or lean body mass (LBM), and your fat.

Our goal is to help you lose FAT instead of WEIGHT, as losing muscle will degrade your health and undermine your ability to keep your weight under control in the long term.

However, this is NOT a body building program. If you want to shed fat, get uber-lean, and build a well defined muscular or "ripped" physique, then we suggest a more rigorous program such as the excellent *Burn the Fat, Feed the Muscle*.

Our emphasis with *The Bipolar Diet* is on the "doable" rather than the "extreme". Yes, it would be ideal if we all attained the bodies of fitness models, but our primary focus is on improving your mental and physical health as much as possible, by using a plan you can stick to for the rest of your life. If you experience rapid success and have a particular passion for fitness, then by all means pursue bigger goals and go for it. On the other hand, it is important to understand that the majority of both your mental and physical gains will be achieved by:

- using the meal plans in Chapter 8 as your main daily guide

- making the Bipolar Super Foods described in Chapter 2 the foundation of your eating plan

- avoiding the Dirty Dozen described in Chapter 3, AND

- aiming to stay within a healthy fat body fat range, without worrying too much about your exact weight in pounds, or reaching the ultra-ripped, fitness model or body builder ideals of uber-low body fat.

How much body fat?

What does all this mean?

For women, the average body fat percentage is 21-25%, whilst a "lean" or "better than average" range would be 16-20%.

For men, the average body fat percentage is 15-19%, whilst a "lean" or "better than average" range would be 10-14%.

We suggest the following target ranges are realistic, achievable, and conducive to excellent health and disease prevention:

For women, a target range of 18-23% body fat.

For men, a target range of 12-17% body fat.

Managing weight vs managing body fat

Your weight and your body fat are closely related, but there are some important differences:

1. Usually if you are "overweight" this excess weight will consist overwhelmingly of excess fat.

2. It is possible to be a suitable weight for your age, height and sex, according to the traditional charts, but still have an unhealthy body

composition with a higher percentage of body fat than is good for you.

3. Losing "weight" may be unhealthy and counter-productive if what you are really losing is muscle instead of fat.

4. It is hard to gain muscle and lose fat at the same time, so concentrate on losing the fat first.

5. The best way to calculate your ideal weight is to base your goal weight on a healthy body fat target range.

For example:

Claire weighs 180 lbs and her body fat is 40%. She decides her first goal should be to get just inside the suggested range, and that she will work towards body fat of 23%. At 180 lbs and 40% body fat, she has a lean muscle weight of 108 lbs, and 72 lbs of fat. She wants to lose fat not muscle, so her goal weight is her existing 108 lbs of lean body mass, PLUS a safer 23% fat, which would be approximately 25 lbs. (108 x .23 = 24.84) For now, her goal weight will be 108 lbs + 25 lbs = 133 lbs.

I currently weigh 157 lbs with 28% body fat. So far I have lost 38 lbs and look and feel much better. However, I decide I want to really go for it, and my target is 19% body fat. My ultimate goal is my existing 113 lbs of muscle plus 19% fat. This equals 113 + (113 x .19 = 21.47). I decide to round it up and be kind to myself, so my long term goal is 113 +22 = 135 lbs.

Calculating your daily calorie requirements

The expert physiologists William McArdle and Frank Katch estimate that the average daily calorie requirements for adults in the US are:

1. 2000 – 2100 calories for women, and

2. 2700 – 2900 calories per day for men.

Many successful weight management programs are based on these general estimates and it is possible to use these figures as the basis for your program, especially if you are of "average" height, weight, build, and activity level.

Obviously to get better results, you should personalize these general guidelines by calculating your individual daily calorie requirements based on your own current weight and body composition (how much of your body is lean muscle mass and how much of it is fat).

The best way to personalize your calculation of the calories you need each day to MAINTAIN your body weight, is by using a simple formula called the Katch-McArdle formula.

There are many different ways of calculating daily calorie requirements, but the Katch-McArdle formula tends to be the most accurate because it is based on lean body mass. Muscle burns more calories than fat, so a more muscular body burns more calories, even at rest, than a body with a higher percentage of body fat.

Instead of bothering with a bunch of complicated formulas and expensive, hard to operate gadgets, I suggest you purchase a set of bathroom scales that provide both total body weight, and body fat percentage. The ones I use are made by Omron and

I purchased them on Amazon for $36.95. They are fantastic! Or of you already have scales you are happy with, you can buy an Omron handheld body fat monitor from Amazon for $26.99. I have one of these as well. It is a nifty device that you simply grasp with both hands to get an accurate measurement of your body fat percentage. I know some experts advocate skin fold tests and so forth but these are hard to perform.

Once you know your body fat percentage and weight, the calculation is easy:

1. Calculate your lean body mass (LBM). This is your total weight, minus the fat. For example, if you weigh 160 lbs, and your body fat percentage is 35%, then your body fat is 160 lbs x .35 = 56, and your LBM = 160 total weight minus 56 lbs of fat = 104 lbs LBM.

   Or, if your weight is 180lbs and your body fat percentage is 40%, then your LBM = (180 x .4 =72), (180 – 72) = 108 lbs LBM.

2. Next we use the formula to calculate your basal metabolic rate (BMR). BMR is simply the amount of energy expended by your body when it is at rest in order to maintain normal bodily functions such as digestion, heartbeat, and respiration. It is expressed in calories.

3. BMR = 370 + (21.6 x LBM in kilograms (kg))

   For example:

   You weigh 155 lbs

   Your body fat percentage is 28% (43.4 lbs fat, 111.6 LBM)

   1 kg = 2.2 lbs

LBM in kg = 111.6 lbs divided by 2.2 = 50.72 kg

Your BMR = 370 + (21.6 X 50.72) = 370 + 1096.2 = 1466 calories

BUT REMEMBER: This is your basal metabolic rate - the calories your body needs at rest. To better estimate the actual number of calories you really need each day, we must also take your activity level into account. So the final step is multiply the BMR calories by activity level:

4. Sedentary (classic desk job with little or no exercise) = BMR x 1.2 activity factor

   Lightly active (light exercise or playing regular sports 1-3 days per week) = BMR X 1.375 activity factor

   Moderately active (moderate exercise or regular sport 3-5 days per week) = BMR X 1.55 activity factor

   Very active (strenuous exercise or vigorous sport 6 days a week) = BMR X 1.725 activity factor

   Extremely Active (daily exercise plus a very physical job, or rigorous all day training such as football camp) = BMT x 1.9 activity factor

Let's pull all this together using my own stats as an example. When I was at most fat and unfit I had really piled on the weight due to the meds I was taking and I got virtually no exercise. My weight ballooned out to 195 lbs and I had a horrifying body fat percentage of 44.9%:

Example 1

My daily calorie needs in order to maintain that same weight:

My weight = 195 lbs

My body fat percentage 44.9% (87.5 lbs fat, 107.5 LBM)

1 kg = 2.2 lbs

LBM in kg = 107.5 lbs divided by 2.2 = 48.86 kg

My old BMR was 370 + (21.6 X 48.86) = 370 + 1055 = 1425 calories

Total daily calorie needs = sedentary 1.2 x 1425 = 1710 daily calories

Next, let's look my new daily calorie needs with a lower body weight, healthier body fat percentage, and regular daily exercise:

Example 1

My daily calorie needs in order to maintain my new, healthier weight:

My weight = 157 lbs

My body fat percentage 28% (44 lbs fat, 113 LBM)

1 kg = 2.2 lbs

LBM in kg = 113 lbs divided by 2.2 = 51.3 kg

My new BMR is 370 + (21.6 X 51.3) = 370 + 1108 = 1478 calories

Total daily calorie needs = moderate 1.55 x 1495 = 2290 daily calories

Some points to note:

- Knowing your individual BMR and daily calorie requirements allows you to create a highly customized, very precise plan for weight management.

- Effective meal planning obviously requires that you know how many calories per day you must consume in order to either gain, lose, or maintain your current weight, depending on your personal health goals.

- As you can see from the figures above, today I can actually eat 600 calories a day more than I could when I was a whopping 38 lbs heavier, WITHOUT gaining weight. This is because of my increased exercise level, but also because I HAVE GAINED MUSCLE.

- The best meal plan will be one that encourages your body to burn fat while preserving, or even building muscle.

- Educate yourself about healthy portion sizes. Portion control is an easy to develop skill based on simple visual cues that empowers you to make smarter choices without missing out on the treats you love.

Chapter 8: Sample Daily Food Plans

Your choice of eating plan will depend on 2 factors:

1. Your daily calorie needs as determined by the formula provided in Chapter 7.

2. Whether you are seeking to lose, gain, or maintain your weight.

And remember – over time your weight, body composition, activity level, and goals will all change, so recalculate your daily calorie needs regularly, and change plans whenever you need to.

Guiding principles

If you have read Chapter 2 on Bipolar Super Foods and Chapter 3 on the "Dirty Dozen", or the 12 foods people with bipolar disorder should almost never eat, then the structure of the meal plans will already make sense to you.

First of all, this is a high protein diet that is designed to make sure you are eating enough lean protein to maximize your mental and physical health. It is not a radically low carb diet like the Atkins Diet and you can have moderate amounts of "good" carbs such as green vegetables. However, "Bad" carbs like refined flour and sugar are definitely to be avoided. The final element is fat. The ideal is to consume less than 37% of your total calories as fat, and healthy fats at that – preferably monosaturated fats such as olive oil. (See the section on saturated fat and trans fat in Chapter 3.) The actual ratio followed is approximate, not strict, and is usually around 35% of your daily calories from protein, 40% from carbs, and 25% from healthy fats.

Of course, everyone needs to bust out and cheat from time to time. We even encourage this as it actually aids fat loss if your body consumes an irregular quantity of calories per day. This prevents your body adjusting to decreased fuel intake and your metabolism from slowing down. BUT you are encouraged to think in terms of a weekly "free meal" or "cheat meal" and NOT a whole "free day" or "cheat day". A whole day is simply too much – it prevents you from really changing your habits and can involve enough extra calories and mood sabotaging sugar and fat to ruin your efforts.

ALSO, please review the section on portion control. The best way to cheat is follow the rules of portion control. This way you can have controlled amounts of the things you love. It will prevent you from feeling deprived and allow your plan to be practical, flexible and easy to stick with, WITHOUT undermining your long term success!

To maintain weight

First, check your body fat and make sure you are happy with your body fat percentage and overall body composition, as well as with your overall weight.

Then all you need to do is calculate your daily calorie needs according to the formula in Chapter 7 and choose the appropriate plan.

Use the Snack Chart at the end of this Chapter 8 in order to fine tune the plan to your exact requirements. For example, if you need 2600 daily calories, base your eating on the 2500 calorie plan and add one extra 100 calorie snack.

However, you should still monitor your weight and body fat, especially in the early days. Some people have faster metabolisms due to lots of muscle or good genetics. Also, some medications contribute to weight loss. Another variable is the activity factor. You may have misjudged how much exercise you are getting and multiplied your BMR by too high or low an activity factor. (This happened to me when I first started treadmilling – my activity felt "moderate", but it was still only "light" until I cranked things up!) All these factors can call for some fine tuning, so check your weight and body fat each week to make sure you are on track.

To lose weight

By now I hope you understand that what this really means is LOSE FAT! This requires keeping up an adequate level of protein, eating plenty of fiber, and getting at least some exercise (see Chapter 9). Above all, it means keeping your metabolism stoked and burning fat by avoiding the "Starvation Response".

The starvation response

It is critical to your success that you be patient and aim for a slow and steady weight loss of 1-2 lbs per week by creating just a small calorie shortfall. If you drastically reduce your food intake, you risk falling victim to the starvation response.

This is an ancient physiological principle that developed when our ancestors were hunting and gathering food many thousands of years ago. Back then there was no such concept as a "diet". Food supply to the body was usually only cut off in times of famine or when game was hard to find. The human body would cope with any sudden reduction in food by going into preservation mode and simply shutting down. Today your body will still respond to a radical food shortage in the same way.

The route to weight loss is a faster metabolism, NOT a slower one, so be patient and don't risk sending your body starvation messages.

Rules for cutting calories

1. NEVER cut calories to below 1200 per day for women and 1800 per day for men. (This guideline comes from the American College of Sports Medicine and is widely recognized by weight loss and fitness experts.)

2. NEVER cut calories by more 1000 calories a day below your daily calorie needs.

3. DO use one of these established rules of thumb for safe, steady weight loss:

    - understanding that 1 pound of fat equates to 3500 calories, and that there are 7 days in a week, cut calories by 500-750 per day. This is a weekly reduction of 3500 – 5250 calories, which will deliver 1-2 lbs of fat loss, especially in combination with regular exercise, OR

    - use the 15-20% rule to really personalize your program and prevent you from falling into the starvation response. For example, if your daily calorie requirements are 1750, cut calories by 20% or 350 calories to 1400 calories per day. (In this example a cut of 500 -750 would reduce daily calories to just 1250 – 1050, which is pretty low and could slow your metabolism too much or result in muscle loss instead of fat loss.)

4. Eat frequent small meals and snacks so that your metabolism remains fired up, despite the reduced fuel.

5. Keep revising your daily calorie needs as your body fat % and activity level change. Losing weight may actually result in switching to a higher calorie food plan so make sure you keep track of your stats and monitor and adjust each week until you reach your goal!

To gain weight

Most people actually need to gain muscle as opposed to fat. Do this by increasing your food intake while still following *The Bipolar Diet* guidelines of high protein, moderate good carbs, low or no bad carbs, and enough good fats. (Actually you will follow APPROXIMATELY a 35:40:25 ratio.)

Concentrate on muscle building resistance exercise such as weight training or resistance bands and do only moderate cardio. (See Chapter 9 for more details on exercise.)

1200 calorie plan

Meal	Calories	Protein	Carb	Fat	Fiber
Breakfast					
Skim Milk (1cup)	80	8g	12g	0g	0g
Scrambled eggs (1 whole, 3 whites)	126	17g	2g	5g	0g
1 slice whole wheat toast	65	5g	9g	1g	2g
1 tablespoon *Smart Balance Omega-3 Light*	50	0g	0g	5g	0g
1 sachet *Metamucil* fiber (sugar free)	20	0g	5g	0g	3g
Snack 1					
Myoplex Lite Chocolate Fudge drink	170	20g	20g	2g	5g
Lunch					
Lean Cuisine Salmon with Basil	220	19g	23g	6g	4g
Snack 2					
Breakstones Live Active Cottage Cheese	90	10g	8g	2g	3g
Dinner					
4 oz grilled chicken breast	155	24g	0g	4g	0g
1 cup broccoli	36	3g	6g	0g	2g
1 cup green beans	34	2g	8g	0g	3g
1/2 cup cooked brown rice	85	1.5g	12g	1g	2g
½ tablespoon olive oil	60	0g	0g	7g	0g
1 sachet *Metamucil* fiber (sugar free)	20	0g	5g	0g	3g
TOTAL	1211	107.5g	102g	33g	27g

Note that this plan has approximately 35% calories from protein, just under 25% calories from fat, and includes extra fiber. Daily fiber intake should be at least 25-30 grams, and so supplements are the easiest way to make sure you are getting enough. Also note that at least 8 glasses of water or other *Bipolar Diet* beverages such as green tea and herb tea should be consumed daily.

1400 calorie plan

Meal	Calories	Protein	Carb	Fat	Fiber
Breakfast *Quakers Instant Oatmeal Weight Control* with 1 scoop *EAS 100% whey protein: chocolate flavor*	280	30g	32g	5g	7g
1 sachet *Metamucil* fiber (sugar free)	20	0g	5g	0g	3g
Snack 1 1 cup fresh blueberries and 4 oz *Publix Cottage Cheese*	195	14g	25g	5g	4g
Lunch *Kashi Southwest Style Chicken* frozen dinner	240	16g	32g	5g	6g
Snack 2 *Kashi Go Lean Roll Bar*	190	12g	28g	5g	6g
Dinner 4 oz grilled salmon	206	29g	0g	5.8g	0g
1 cup broccoli	36	3g	6g	0g	2g
1 small (6oz) baked potato	157	3g	36g	0g	3g
1 tablespoon *Smart Balance Omega-3 Light*	50	0g	0g	5g	0g
1 sachet *Metamucil* fiber (sugar free)	20	0g	5g	0g	3g
TOTAL	1394	107g	169g	30.8	34g

Note that this is a higher carb/lower fat plan, with approximately 31% calories from protein, 48% calories from carbs, and 21% calories from fat. It is also very high fiber. This is a good plan for women who want to stay nicely above the 1200 daily minimum and get things moving, but who want to limit their lean protein and not restrict carbs too much.

As a low calorie plan, it would be unsuitable for anyone who is highly active or very overweight. Ideally calories should be just enough to create a daily deficit of 500-750 calories, or by 15-20% of daily needs as calculated using the formula in Chapter 7.

And remember - at least 8 glasses of water or other *Bipolar Diet* beverages such as green tea and herb tea should be consumed daily.

1800 calorie plan

Meal	Calories	Protein	Carb	Fat	Fiber
Breakfast					
1 egg (boiled, poached, scrambles or fried non-stick) with 1 slice *Nature's Own Double Fiber*	130	10g	11g	4.5g	5g
Wheat toast and 1 tablespoon *Smart Balance Omega-3 Light*	50	0g	0g	5g	0g
1 cup *Kashi Go Lean* cereal with 150g *Fage Total Nonfat* Greek style yoghurt	220	26g	36g	1g	10g
Snack 1					
Hass Avocado	83	1g	4g	7g	3g
Breakstones Live Active Cottage Cheese	90	10g	8g	2g	3g
Lunch					
Sandwich made from 2 slices of *Ezekiel 4:9 Sprouted Grain* bread, filled with 3 oz grilled chicken breast, grated carrot, romaine lettuce and tomato. *(*Grill your chicken at home by rubbing boneless and skinless breasts with olive oil, salt and pepper and herbs taste – rosemary, oregano, paprika – whatever you prefer. This is much better for you and cheaper than buying the precooked kind.) For a healthy dressing use ½ tablespoon olive oil.	328	21g	33g	12g	7g
Snack 2					
Myoplex Lite Chocolate Fudge drink	170	20g	20g	2g	5g
Dinner					
4 oz Ahi tuna steak	140	33.7g	0g	1.3g	0g
10 asparagus spears	40	4g	6g	0g	3g
1 small (6oz) baked potato	157	3g	36g	0g	3g
1 tablespoon *Smart Balance Omega-3 Light*	50	0g	0g	5g	0g
Jell-O Sugar-Free Dark Chocolate 1 pudding	60	2g	12g	1g	0g
Hood Simply Smart milk (fat free) (1cup)	90	10g	13g	0g	0g

Meal	Calories	Protein	Carb	Fat	Fiber
Snack 3 *Healthy Choice Chicken with Rice* soup	180	12g	26g	3g	4g
TOTAL	1788	144g	205g	44g	43g

This is an interesting plan with 32% calories from protein, 46% calories from carbs, and 22% calories from fat. As you can see, a third snack is included now that the overall daily calorie allowance is getting higher. It is better for your mood stability and weight control to eat regular small meals instead of just 2-3 really big ones. It also has plenty of fiber! As usual, plenty of water and herbal tea should also be consumed.

2000 calorie plan

Meal	Calories	Protein	Carb	Fat	Fiber
Breakfast 1 Thomas' Hearty Grain Whole Wheat Bagel	240	10g	49g	2g	7g
3oz fat free cream cheese	90	12g	6g	0g	0g
1 sachet Metamucil fiber (sugar free)	20	0g	5g	0g	3g
Snack 1 Kashi Go Lean Roll Bar	190	12g	28g	5g	6g
Lunch Crispers chef salad, dressed with 1 tablespoon olive oil. Season with sea salt.	510	40g	12g	25g	3g
Snack 2 Myoplex Lite Chocolate Fudge drink	170	20g	20g	2g	5g
Dinner Stir fry with 1 cup brown rice (cooked),	160	4g	34g	1g	2g
1 cup mixed stir fry oriental vegetables, and	50	2g	9g	0g	2g
5 oz extra lean sirloin cut into strips.	286	43g	0g	11g	0g
Hood Simply Smart milk (fat free) (1cup)	90	10g	13g	0g	0g
1 sachet Metamucil fiber (sugar free)	20	0g	5g	0g	3g
Snack 3 170g Fage Total Nonfat Greek style yoghurt (1 container) with 1 cup blueberries	174	16g	28g	0g	4g
TOTAL	2000	181g	209g	46g	

This plan features approximately 36% calories from protein, 42% calories from carbs, and 21% calories from fat.

Despite the high quantity of fat in the Crispers salad, by being careful with all the other day's choices the overall ratio works out well.

Alternative 2000 calorie plan

Meal	Calories	Protein	Carb	Fat	Fiber
Breakfast *Kelloggs' Special K Protein Plus* cereal with 1 cup *Hood Simply Smart milk* (fat free)	190	20g	27g	3g	0g
1 tablespoon *MaraNatha Creamy Almond Butter* with 1 slice *Nature's Own Whitewheat* toast	130	6.5g	14g	8.5g	4.5g
"Jaffa shake" with 1 scoop *Jay Robb Egg White Protein Chocolate Flavor Powder* and 1 sachet orange *Metamucil* fiber (sugar free)	140	24g	9g	0g	3g
Snack 1 *Healthy Choice Chicken with Rice* soup	180	12g	26g	3g	4g
Lunch Kashi Lime Cilantro Shrimp	250	12g	33g	8g	6g
Kashi Go Lean Roll Bar	190	12g	28g	5g	6g
Snack 2 *Myoplex Lite Chocolate Fudge* drink	170	20g	20g	2g	5g
Dinner 4 oz grilled salmon	206	29g	0g	5.8g	0g
1 cup green beans	34	2g	8g	0g	3g
1 small (6oz) baked potato with 1 tablespoon	157	3g	36g	0g	3g
Smart Balance Omega-3 Light	50	0g	0g	5g	0g
2 cups mixed green salad with 3 tablespoon light Italian dressing	52	0g	10g	0g	5g
Jell-O Sugar-Free Dark Chocolate 1 pudding	60	2g	12g	1g	0g
Snack 3 1 cup fresh blueberries and 4 oz *Publix Cottage Cheese*	195	14g	25g	5g	4g
TOTAL	2004	156.5g	248g	46.3g	37g

This alternative plan is higher in carbs relative to protein and features approximately 30% calories from protein, 49% calories from carbs, and 21% calories from fat. Note the use of egg white protein as an excellent protein powder that can be made into shakes and so forth for people who do not want to consume milk products. It has no fat and virtually no carbs. **NOTE THAT THE SAMPLE PLANS ALL FEATURE SOME PRE-PACKAGED FOODS SUCH AS FROZEN MEALS, SOUPS, PROTEIN SHAKES AND SO FORTH.** Cooking fresh food from scratch is cheaper and healthier but we have included these convenience foods in the interests of practicality, to help get you started and in the belief that these are still better than junk foods with much higher amounts of simple "bad" carbs and saturated fats and/or trans fats.

Snack Chart & Custom Menu Planner

Food	Calories	Protein	Carb	Fat	Fiber
Skim Milk (1cup)	80	8g	12g	0g	0g
Hood Simply Smart milk (fat free) (1cup)	90	10g	13g	0g	0g
Jaffa shake with 1 cup fat free *Hood Smart Milk,* 1 sachet orange *Metamucil* fiber, 1 scoop *EAS 100% whey protein: chocolate flavor*	230	33g	21g	2g	4g
12 Almonds	80	3g	3g	7g	1.5g
Hass Avocado	83	1g	4g	7g	3g
Boiled egg	80	6g	1g	4.5g	0g
Teriyaki Beef Jerky (1 oz)	80	12g	6g	1g	0g
Cracker Barrel 2% Cheddar Cheese Stick	90	7g	1g	6g	0g
Stonyfield Farm fat free plain yoghurt	80	8g	12g	0g	0g
Myoplex Lite Chocolate Fudge drink	170	20g	20g	2g	5g
Breakstones Live Active Cottage Cheese	90	10g	8g	2g	3g
Lean Cuisine Salmon with Basil	220	19g	23g	6g	4g
Healthy Choice Chicken with Rice soup	180	12g	26g	3g	4g
Quakers Instant Oatmeal	280	30g	32g	5g	7g

The Bipolar Diet

Food	Calories	Protein	Carb	Fat	Fiber
Weight Control with 1 scoop *EAS 100% whey protein: chocolate flavor*					
1 can *King Oscar Sardines* (in spring water) and 1 slice *Martins 100% Whole Wheat Potato Bread*	140	19g	14g	11g	4g
1 egg (boiled, poached, scrambles or fried non-stick) with 1 slice *Nature's Own Double Fiber Wheat* toast	130	10g	11g	4.5g	5g
1 tablespoon *MaraNatha Creamy Almond Butter* with 1 slice *Nature's Own Whitewheat* toast	130	6.5g	14g	8.5g	4.5g
4 oz *Publix Cottage Cheese* and 1 *Thomas' Hearty Double Fiber English* muffin	221	18g	31g	5.5g	5g
1 cup fresh blueberries and 4 oz *Publix Cottage Cheese*	195	14g	25g	5g	4g
1 cup *Kashi Go Lean* cereal with 150g *Fage Total Nonfat* Greek style yoghurt	220	26g	36g	1g	10g
Jell-O Sugar-Free Dark Chocolate 1 pudding	60	2g	12g	1g	0g
Kashi Go Lean Roll Bar	190	12g	28g	5g	6g
Planters Pistachio Lovers Mix 35 pieces, 28g	160	6g	7g	13g	3g
Earthharvest Pumpkorn shelled pumpkin seeds, dry roasted	140	9g	4g	11g	1g

Food	Calories	Protein	Carb	Fat	Fiber
with organic seasoning, 28 g					
5 oz strawberries (about 8 medium sized) and ½ cup whipped cream topping (pressurized) (no sugar)	122	2g	13g	6.5g	4g

Chapter 9:
The Truth About Exercise

Sometimes it feels like they are doing it just to annoy us – it seems like everywhere you turn, someone is trumpeting the value of exercise. Don't these people know I HATE to exercise? Don't they know I have heard it all before, and I would do it if I could? That I am too depressed? Too anxious? Too distracted? Too busy? Too fat or self-conscious?

Believe me, I am not bringing up exercise just to press your buttons.

I was one of those folks who hated exercise and generally avoided it, except for a couple of things like long leisurely walks and riding my bicycle – as long as the weather was not too hot, not too cold, not too windy, not threatening rain – I am sure you get the picture.

After a couple of years of nagging from my doctor, my shrink, and my loved ones, I decided exercise may be worth trying after all. I had stacked on 40 lbs of unattractive fat from various medications, my moods were starting to destabilize, and I had some very scary cholesterol and other test results that made it pretty clear that both my mental and my physical health were seriously compromised. Plus, my clothes didn't fit, and I pretty much hated myself.

Also, I had started a serious, intense study of bipolar disorder and nutrition, and over and over again the same studies and textbooks that explained the benefits of *The Bipolar Diet* also revealed convincing evidence that exercise had profound benefits for people with bipolar disorder –even more so than for members of the general public.

So I gave it a try . . . and what I have discovered has changed my life!

The benefits of exercise

In their textbook, *Manic-Depressive Illness: Bipolar Disorders and Recurrent Depression,* Drs Goodwin and Jamison describe two of the greatest benefits of exercise for people with bipolar disorder:

1. Powerful anti-depressant effect.

2. When done at the same time each day it synchronizes the circadian clock and thus powerfully contributes to overall mood and mental stability.

For me, I believe exercise has also been one the biggest factors in rebuilding my self-respect. I was someone who had serious guilt and shame issues arising from the dreadful things I had done when highly manic or depressed. The boost I got from pursuing exercise as a kind of "self-treatment", where I could see substantial benefits compounding, all due entirely to my own efforts, was huge!

And of course, if one of your goals in following *The Bipolar Diet* is weight loss, then exercise is critical. In fact, all 3 of the goals of *The Bipolar Diet* are greatly enhanced through regular exercise.

Another plus is that exercise elevates mood without inducing mania. For anyone who misses the euphoria, and enhanced powers of creativity, focus, and achievement that come with the "up" side of the roller coaster, exercise can help you recapture all the positives, WITHOUT risking a manic episode. In fact, it will promote mood stability, but with a wonderful "calm energy" that is much better than the jittery high of drugs, caffeine, or acute mania.

- Natural anti-depressant
- Improve heart health
- Improve insulin response
- Lower cholesterol
- Lower blood pressure
- Stay young and flexible
- Stable circadian rhythm (body clock) for increased mood stability
- Lose weight
- Sleep better
- Improve digestion
- Increase energy
- Explode self-respect.

I was able to brainstorm this list of 12 benefits of exercise in under a minute, without stopping to really even think. There are probably 100 reasons to exercise – 101 for those of us who are bipolar.

What type of exercise?

There are only a couple of guidelines you need to follow when deciding on the type of exercise:

1. It must be aerobic.

2. It must be performed at roughly the same time each day in order to reap the benefits of improved circadian rhythms.

3. Don't exercise last thing at night. Schedule your exercise sessions to be finished at least 3 hours before bedtime.

Wait a minute . . . did you just say I have to take up aerobics? No! Don't worry! Aerobic exercise simply means any exercise that is strenuous enough to increase your need for oxygen. This can be brisk walking, jogging, dancing, cycling, swimming, jumping rope, and so on – anything that uses your large muscle groups and gets your heart rate up. Things like Tai Chi or yoga also provide great benefits and have a place in your wellness program, but what we are talking about here is something that really gets your blood pumping!

If your heart and lungs are working harder than usual for an extended period, then whatever you are doing is probably aerobic exercise. (And of course, if you are someone who loves music and dance and the buzz of group activity, then by all means DO take up aerobics ☺)

How much exercise?

The minimum should be a twenty minute walk, most days of the week.

However, when it comes to exercise more effort always equals greater rewards. To get truly powerful anti-depressant or weight loss effects you need to do more than the minimum.

Although a daily walk will definitely improve your moods and your physical health, a more vigorous and extended workout will yield far more dramatic rewards, so the extra effort is more than worth it.

These days, I exercise 6 days a week. I alternate longer walking sessions on the treadmill (90 minutes so I can watch two episodes of a favorite show such as Lost or Desperate Housewives) with shorter, more strenuous sessions of jogging for 30 -40 minutes.

OK – but I REALLY HATE to exercise . . .

For me, getting past the barriers meant looking carefully at what I didn't like about exercise and coming up with a custom plan that was tailored to overcome all my pet excuses:

- I am a "head" person and exercise is boring
- I live in Florida and it is just too hot
- I am self-conscious and don't want people sniggering at me at the gym
- There is nothing I am good at
- And blah blah blah!

Today this all seems so whiney and petty, but that is where I was at. My solution was to invest in a treadmill and exercise in the privacy of my home with the A/C cranked up, and some great DVDs to watch. As the weight dropped off, my moods and energy soared, and the exercise became first a habit and then a pleasure, I started cranking up the intensity and now often ditch the DVDs so I can focus on working out to the best of my ability.

Boxing, martial arts, hiking, tennis? Try to think of something you have enjoyed in the past. Everyone can walk, so walk –even if it takes an exercise buddy or an iPod to get past the tedium. Another great way to get going is Wii exercise. Their latest exercise games are a blast.

- A good alternative to DVDs on the treadmill is reading on a stationary bike.
- If you hate getting sweaty try aqua-aerobics.
- If you would rather be shopping, buy cool sneakers and sexy work-out clothes.
- If the whole idea completely pisses you off, buy a heavy bag and some boxing gloves.

Once you get started the rewards help supply motivation, but in the beginning, finding something fun and having moral support are critical.

It also helps to take up some active hobbies and incorporate exercise into your daily routine. We go hiking, geocaching, or bird watching most Sundays, and on work days I follow all the usual tips – taking the stairs, parking further away from the store, always doing one active chore like vacuuming or mowing the lawn or weeding a flowerbed.

Inertia is almost impossible to overcome, but once you get some momentum going, climbing the mountain changes to freewheeling downhill.

That is why our next chapter is all about getting and staying motivated . . .

Chapter 10:
Staying Motivated

PLEASE my friends, do NOT sit around waiting for motivation to strike.

I once read somewhere that there is no point working on "self-esteem" because it is a feeling, and is therefore temporary, erratic and unreliable – kind of like weather. Instead, it is better to focus on something more concrete like "self-respect", and to do something tangible and specific every day that will build self-respect. For example, keeping a promise to yourself, doing a good deed, learning a new skill, sticking to your food plan, and so forth.

Motivation is much the same. It does not magically show up out of the blue, so don't waste time or risk your health by sitting around and waiting for it. BUT if you start taking action, BEFORE you feel motivated, then you will find that little by little your motivation will increase.

There is no magic bullet that I can pass on through this book. YOU MUST MAKE YOUR OWN DECISION that NOW is the time to improve your mental, emotional, and physical health through better diet and exercise habits.

Keep your focus on how much better you can manage your bipolar symptoms and mood swings, and thereby improve every aspect of your life. This should be your ultimate goal.

However, some people do better when they have a series of mini-goals or more specific motivators. Let me explain . . .

Baby steps

Almost everything is easier when we break it down into baby steps. For me, knowing I needed to lose over 40lbs was an overwhelming feeling. But losing 5 lbs? No Worries! I used monthly mini goals of 5 lbs a month and planned out my menus, exercise routine, and calorie requirements in advance. (Remember, your weight, body fat%, and your activity level will be changing as your program progresses, so re-assessing every month is ideal.)

Carrot and stick

For specific motivators, you can use a carrot and stick approach – first the carrot - rewards for achieving your goals. My reward system consisted of things that reinforced my improved appearance and self-confidence such as a new blouse or purse or a pedicure. In my less shallow moments, I love to read, so some months my reward is to treat myself to something off my Amazon wish list.

As for the "stick" – for me it was easy to get motivated through the fear factor. My father died of a heart attack when he was 46, and my grandmother also died in her 40s, so I knew I couldn't afford to stall if I wanted to avoid an early death. I also worked myself into a terror of diabetes. This is a very realistic fear if you are overweight, especially if you have bipolar disorder. I would imagine worst case scenarios like going blind or having a leg amputated – a treadmill session along with

"Desperate Housewives" is not really hard to face in comparison!

Get a buddy

Why does the buddy system work, and why does it work so well? Perhaps the number one reason is that it helps you make a commitment. If you promise a trusted friend that you will walk with him or her every weekend morning at 8 am (or play tennis, or go golfing, etc.), if you are a good friend you will probably feel some sort of pull to fulfill this commitment. So basically, the buddy system puts positive pressure on you to go carry out your exercise plans.

Another reason is that the right buddy makes exercise fun again. The perfect exercise partner is not just reliable and consistent – they are someone you admire, feel close to, and whose company you always enjoy. Ideally, your exercise partner will be at a similar physical level so that you never feel pressured to under- or over-perform. Walking and talking with someone important to you is always worthwhile and accomplishing goals together will cement the relationship and make it even stronger.

Avoiding sabotage

If you have a friend that always want to eat fast food or go get ice cream and tells you that it's ok to cheat on your diet "just this once" or says other things that disparage your efforts, don't hang out with that person anymore.

Don't expect that person to support you in your weight loss goal and find a new friend who will go work out with you, eat healthy with you, and help you stay motivated to lose weight. Losing weight can be a real struggle and it's important to have some strong, supportive friends who will support you because they love you and want you to be healthy.

Sometimes, friends can be jealous when one friend starts to really improve their lives by getting a new job or losing weight. Unfortunately, you might have to be willing not to spend time with that person anymore in order to accomplish your goals.

If your family is not supportive of your desire to get healthy because it means they have to give up junk food or other foods, don't let them derail you. Stand firm and tell them if they want junk food to eat it outside the house or buy their own and keep it in their rooms.

Don't let anyone hold you back from doing what you know is best for you – making healthy food choices and getting the exercise you need!

A few months ago, the media was all over a story about weight gain being contagious. Your health is intimately connected to the people around you, and ideally you AND your loved ones will all value a healthy mind in a healthy body for the whole family.

Kick excuses to the curb

See your excuses for what they really are – empty justifications for not fulfilling our obligations. The surest way to build motivation is to build self-respect, and the surest way to build self-respect is to DROP THE EXCUSES! We have all heard them a million times:

- Not enough time
- Too many family obligations

- You can't afford to join the gym
- Exercise is no fun
- Fill in the blank _____!

The truth is that ALL of the millions of people who exercise regularly and organize healthy meals for themselves and their families have the same 24 hours in the day that you do. As for family obligations, taking care of yourself is a MAJOR obligation you have to your family. The About.com Exercise webpage has this advice for folks who are using their family as an excuse:

> *"You don't have to neglect your family to fit in exercise. Join a health club that has a daycare center or do a video while they nap. If they're old enough, have them participate in your routine by lifting very small weights or counting your repetitions, or take them with you on your daily walk. Show your family what it means to be healthy by giving them a good role model."*

You can accomplish all the health goals of *The Bipolar Diet* with a daily walk. Sure, join the gym if that is what you enjoy and find motivating, but if you cannot afford it, it is NOT a necessity.

Most excuses below in the same category. Ask yourself – is this an insurmountable obstacle so grounded in reality that nobody could overcome it – or is it an empty justification or avoidance technique that is covering up another issue? (For example, do I have some investment in staying unwell?)

Have a little faith

Research shows that people who regularly attend some place of worship and who live a spiritual lifestyle can be healthier and live longer than their societal counterparts who do not engage in worship activities.

Whether these people live healthier lives because they are following the rules set forth by their place of worship or if it is because they are more at peace than other people as a result of their faith, you should know that actively engaging in some form of worship is generally considered to be one way to live a healthier and more satisfying life.

This is certainly not to say that people who do not engage in some form of worship live empty lives, but if you have an interest in some form of spiritualism then now is the time to hop in and see if a certain place of worship is a good fit for your beliefs.

Not only can you increase your socialization exponentially but you may be able to find more peace in your daily existence depending upon what place of worship you choose to attend.

Effective goal setting

Why are some people so much better at reaching their goals than others? There is a science and a magic to setting goals. Follow these steps:

- Make it concrete, specific and measurable
- Set a timeframe
- Follow a plan
- Track your progress
- Write it down
- Visualize your success: use lots of details and FEEL as well as think
- Begin it now!

Sources and Further Information

Bipolar disorder books:

Of course today there are many excellent choices available so I will just list my two all time favorites. These complement each other nicely as the first is highly technical, but is the most comprehensive and authoritative textbook available (read this and you will know more than your doctor), and the second is deliberately designed for "easy reading" but has terrific content:

Frederick K. Goodwin and Kay Redfield Jamison, *Manic-Depressive Illness: Bipolar Disorders and Recurrent Depression,* 2nd ed, Oxford University Press, 2007.

Candida Fink, MD and Joe Kraynak, *Bipolar Disorder for Dummies,* Wiley Publishing, Inc., 2005

Food and mood books:

Robert E. Thayer, *Calm Energy*, Oxford University Press, 2003.

Jack Challem, *The Food-Mood Solution*, John Wiley & Sons, Inc., 2007.

Elizabeth Somer, *Food & Mood: The Complete Guide to Eating Well and Feeling Your Best*, 2nd ed, Henry Holt and Company, 1999.

Thyroid book:

Although bipolar disorder is not discussed directly, this is an excellent resource that clearly explains symptoms, treatment, and the confusion surrounding what "normal" levels of thyroid hormone really are.

Richard L. Shames and Karilee Halo Shames, *Thyroid Power: 10 Steps to Total Health,* Collins Wellness, 2005.

MUST HAVE books for smart shopping and weight control:

David Zinczenko with Matt Goulding, *Eat This, Not That: Supermarket Survival Guide*, Rodale Inc, 2009.

David Zinczenko with Matt Goulding, *Eat This, Not That! Thousands of Simple Food Swaps That Can Save You 10, 20, 30 Pounds – or More!* Rodale Inc, 2007.

Great Links:

Information about bipolar disorder and increased risk of death and illness

Bipolar Disorder Increases Risk for Premature Death from Medical Illness at http://www.medscape.com/viewarticle/587962

General information about bipolar disorder and nutrition

DBSA (Depression and Bipolar Support Alliance): *Food and Mood* at http://www.dbsalliance.org/pdfs/foodmoode2.pdf

Food for the brain: bipolar disorder at http://www.foodforthebrain.org/content.asp?id_Content=1713

Prevention Magazine: *Bipolar Disorder and Complementary Medicine* at http://www.prevention.com/cda/vendorarticle/bipolar-disorder/HN1167002/health/conditions.treatments/

General information about supplements

Consumer Reports Health.org: Common Natural Medicines

National Institute of Health (NIH): Dietary Supplement Fact Sheets

Mayo Clinic: Herbs, supplements and vitamins

Information about amino acids and bipolar

About.com: Amino acid nutrition and bipolar disorder

Information about fish oil (omega-3) and bipolar

Harvard Medical School: Omega 3 fatty acids in bipolar disorder

British Journal of Psychiatry: Efficacy of EPA in bipolar depression

Journal of Clinical Psychiatry: Omega-3 in bipolar depression

Black Dog Institute: Omega-3 and mood disorders

Information about folic acid, B12 and bipolar

Journal of Psychopharmacology: Folic acid and B12 for Depression

Journal of Affective Disorders: Reduced red-cell folate in mania

Baylor University Medical Center: Folate, vitamin B12, and neuropsychiatric disorders

Information about inositol and bipolar

University of Pittsburgh School of Medicine: Inositol as an add-on treatment for bipolar depression

Ben Gurion University: Inositol for Depression, Panic, and OCD

Interview with Robert Belmaker: Using inositol for promoting brain wellness

Townsend Letter for Doctors & Patients: Low inositol diet for bipolar disorder

Support Groups

About.com Bipolar Disorder provide a weight loss support forum with many high quality resources and additional information that will educate and motivate you.

bp Magazine (an excellent quarterly magazine about bipolar disorder which I highly recommend) has an online forum, which includes a support group for people interested in bipolar disorder and weight management.

Bonus 1: Special Report on Diabetes and Bipolar Disorder

Diabetes and bipolar disorder are comorbid conditions. This means they often coexist, with many people having both bipolar disorder AND diabetes.

Research indicates that this is more than an unfortunate coincidence. Some studies have shown people with bipolar disorder are up to THREE TIMES more likely to have diabetes than members of the general population.

Also, there is evidence that people with bipolar disorder and diabetes are more likely to face other health challenges such as being more prone to rapid cycling, and more likely to have chronic, as opposed to milder, mood episodes. There may be other negative lifestyle consequences as well. One Canadian study found that 81% of bipolar people with diabetes were receiving disability payments, versus 30% of bipolar patients without diabetes.

ALL PEOPLE DIAGNOSED WITH BIPOLAR DISORDER SHOULD IMMEDIATELY HAVE A COMPREHENSIVE PHYSICAL EXAM TO CHECK FOR THE PRESENCE OF COMMOM COMORBID CONDITIONS, ESPECIALLY DIABETES.

What is diabetes?

Diabetes is a disease in which:

- the pancreas no longer produces enough insulin, or

- when cells stop responding to the insulin that is produced,

so that glucose (sugar) in the blood cannot be absorbed into the cells of the body.

In other words, because of either a shortage of insulin, or an inability by the body to make use of insulin, sugar and other food can no longer be correctly metabolized and turned into energy. Sugar simply continues to accumulate in the blood, causing a variety of health problems.

The symptoms of this excess sugar in the bloodstream include:

- frequent urination
- excessive thirst
- physical lethargy
- mental fatigue
- hunger
- blurred vision
- bad breath
- rapid deep breathing
- irritability, anger, or hostility.

(Note that the diabetic mood swings resulting from excess sugar and carbohydrates in the body are extremely similar to the mood swings experienced in bipolar disorder. A person with diabetes may seem depressed, or manic, or both.)

Types of diabetes

Type 1 Diabetes: Formerly called juvenile diabetes or insulin-dependent diabetes, this is usually first diagnosed in children, teenagers or young adults. Treatment for type 1 diabetes includes taking insulin shots or using an insulin pump, making wise food choices, exercising regularly, controlling blood pressure and cholesterol, and islet cell transplantation (an experimental method to help control blood glucose levels without insulin injections).

Type 2 Diabetes: Formerly called adult-onset or non-insulin-dependent diabetes, this is the most common form of diabetes. People can develop type 2 diabetes at any age. Being overweight and inactive increases the chances of developing type 2 diabetes. Treatment includes taking diabetes medicines, making wise food choices, exercising regularly, taking aspirin daily, controlling blood pressure and cholesterol, and use of oral or injected insulin.

Gestational Diabetes: Some women develop gestational diabetes during the late stages of pregnancy. Although this form of diabetes usually goes away after the baby is born, a woman who has had it is more likely to develop type 2 diabetes later in life.

There is also pre-diabetes, which some experts consider America's largest healthcare epidemic. Also known as Syndrome X or metabolic syndrome, this condition occurs when a person's blood glucose levels are higher than normal but not high enough for a diagnosis of type 2 diabetes. As of 2009 there are 57 million Americans who have pre-diabetes.

Bipolar meds and diabetes

Several medications used to treat bipolar disorder can cause significant weight gain, insulin resistance, and hyperglycemia. The drug most associated with contributing to diabetes is Zyprexa. Seroquel and Risperdal have also been linked to the development of diabetes. Ask your doctor if you can try the bipolar medications that don't cause pre-diabetes (metabolic syndrome) first. If you are concerned about metabolic syndrome, it makes sense to only take those drugs likely to cause it if the other bipolar medications prove ineffective for you in treating your bipolar disorder.

Risk factors

The major risk factor for type 1 diabetes is still unknown, although family history appears to play a role.

According to the Mayo Clinic, the risk factors for type 2 diabetes are:

- "**Weight.** *The more fatty tissue you have, the more resistant your cells become to insulin.*
- **Inactivity.** *The less active you are, the greater your risk. Physical activity helps you control your weight, uses up glucose as energy and makes your cells more sensitive to insulin.*
- **Family history.** *Your risk increases if a parent or sibling has type 2 diabetes.*
- **Race.** *Although it's unclear why, people of certain races — including blacks, Hispanics, American Indians and Asian-Americans — are at higher risk.*
- **Age.** *Your risk increases as you get older, especially after age 45. Often, that's because you tend to exercise less, lose muscle mass and gain*

weight as you age. But type 2 diabetes is increasing dramatically among children, adolescents and younger adults.

- **Gestational diabetes.** *If you developed gestational diabetes when you were pregnant, your risk of developing prediabetes and type 2 diabetes later increases. If you gave birth to a baby weighing more than 9 pounds (4 kilograms), you're also at risk of type 2 diabetes.*
- **Polycystic ovary syndrome.** *For women, having polycystic ovary syndrome — a common condition characterized by irregular menstrual periods, excess hair growth and obesity — increases the risk of diabetes."* (See the Mayo Clinic's excellent diabetes section.)

We can also add taking medications such as Zyprexa to this list.

Why do diabetes and bipolar co-occur?

This question has yet to be answered definitively. However, there are several theories, including the following:

- The stress hormone cortisol tends to be elevated in both bipolar patients and diabetics. In particular, very high level levels of cortisol have been observed in people suffering from bipolar depression. Too much cortisol leads to insulin resistance so it is possible that the elevated cortisol in people with bipolar disorder leads to diabetes.

- People with bipolar disorder often self-medicate with food, including the "comfort foods" high in sugar and saturated fats that contribute to both metabolic syndrome and type 2 diabetes.

Treatments

Diabetes is usually treated by changes in diet and through medication, for example regular injections of insulin.

The most important dietary changes are to opt for foods high in nutrition but low in calories, sugar and fat. As stabilizing blood sugar is so important, it is ideal if you can eat your meals at the same time every day, and consume a healthy proportion of carbohydrates, proteins and fats, with little variation to the ratio from day to day.

Increased physical activity such as the kind of exercise program outlined in *The Bipolar Diet* is also important in both treating and preventing metabolic syndrome and type 2 diabetes.

Summary of the bipolar/diabetes connection

Diabetes is a very serious health condition that is a leading cause of death and disability. People with bipolar disorder are more likely to develop diabetes than members of the general population. Further, certain medications used in treating bipolar disorder can induce diabetes. However, the same healthy diet and exercise program that can both prevent and treat type 2 diabetes is also highly effective in treating the symptoms of bipolar.

Bonus 2: Top 6 Techniques for Managing Moods

1. Goal Setting

What does goal setting have to do with mood swings? Everything!

Depression: Goal setting is beneficial during episodes of depression because it encourages a focus on the future; on accomplishments, progress, and positive outcomes; and, when used in the right way, develops problem solving and communication skills.

Mania: Goal setting is also beneficial during bouts of mania, and particularly when on the cusp of developing a manic episode. Mania is often characterized by grandiosity and unrealistic thinking. When done in the manner we will describe, goal setting can encourage reality checks, and the breaking of large schemes into smaller, manageable chunks. Even if the goal is exposed as unrealistic, it is still constructive as it short circuits future frustration, anger, and disappointment, and allows energy to be channeled towards more achievable and constructive projects.

What do we mean by "the right way" to set goals? Many experts advocate the use of the SMART goal setting technique:

Specific **M**easurable **A**chievable **R**ealistic **T**imebound

Specific and measurable goals should be formulated so that you have a precise, concrete and quantifiable target so that you will know when you get there.

Achievable and realistic goals are important so you don't waste energy and resources on something that is impossible or not worthwhile.

You will need to ask questions about:

- what possible problems may be encountered
- the action you must take and how to break things down into a logical plan, and
- what help you will need.

The ideal is to go through this process with friends, family, loved ones, colleagues, or other members of your wellness team.

For a depressed person this reduces isolation and fosters feelings of being supported and connected.

For a manic person, this can provide a very important reality check!

The timebound aspect is the final piece.

You can plan for a week, a month, a year, or even a five year plan. Or, if it is a difficult time when depression or lack of focus is overwhelming, your timeframe may be day by day.

SMART goal setting can be applied to any area of your life:

- self
- relationships
- work
- finances
- navigating change
- health improvement goals, especially weight loss, or starting an exercise program.

2. Try a Little Kindness . . .

One of the universe's greatest paradoxes is the way we end up ultimately helping ourselves whenever we reach out in kindness to help another.

I am not just talking about "karma" here. I mean the measurable, demonstrable real world benefits that flow from being of service to others, especially for those of us with bipolar disorder.

Let me explain . . .

Kindness to others:

- Builds self-respect (which is often damaged by the things we do during episodes of mania or depression)
- Promotes feelings of connectedness and reduces isolation and loneliness
- Reminds us we can also be kind to ourselves
- Shifts our focus from our own moods, thoughts and feelings, which may be unhealthy or fixated, and diverts them to something external and real

- Broadens and deepens our perspective as we practice compassion and get a chance to walk in someone else's shoes.

It is possible to take a daily "kindness inventory". DBSA suggest asking:

- Was I selfish or unkind today?
- Do I owe an apology?
- Have I kept something secret that I need to talk with someone about?
- Was I thinking of myself all day, or did I think of others?
- How can I be kinder tomorrow?

3. Avoid Stressors

Stress plays a major role in bipolar disorder. Although we know that bipolar disorder has a genetic basis and tends to run in families, studies of identical twins show frequent examples of one twin developing bipolar disorder when the other does not. Many experts believe that it is stress – and our response to it – that makes the difference.

I know from keeping my own mood charts that episodes of both mania and depression can be triggered by stressful events in my life, especially if I respond inappropriately.

Here are 10 tips from the Black Dog Institute, a leading bipolar disorder research organization, to help you manage the stress in your life:

Work out priorities: Keep a list of "doable" priorities.

Identify your stressors: What leaves YOU emotionally drained?

Think before you commit yourself to other people's priorities!

Move on: Don't dwell on mistakes. Regret won't change the past.

Express and discuss feelings: Defuse frustration – don't bottle it.

Set aside time each day for recreation and exercise!

Take your time: Don't let people rush you as this leads to stress, mistakes and regrets. Plan ahead and always factor in a buffer of time.

1. **Opt out of road rage:** Don't be an aggressive driver.

2. **Think positively:** You get what you expect, so smile and take the high road.

3. **Avoid drinking, smoking, sedatives and stimulants:** Focus on long term solutions instead of quick fixes that actually make things worse. Treat your physical and mental health as the most important thing in the world, because you know what? It is!

4. Speed Relaxation

Ok, I know it sounds like a contradiction. But sometimes we need to calm down – fast!

It would be great to have long, leisurely relaxation sessions, but sometimes we need a quick and effective technique that we can summon up when we feel stress starting to overwhelm us.

These are techniques that you can even use for just a couple of minutes in the workplace. Remember, everyone is different so don't worry if they don't all work for you. Find one or two that you really like and can master, and use them anytime you need to replace fear and tension with peace and calm:

- Tense your whole body, clenching every muscle as tight as you can. Hold it for as long as you can, then let everything go. Repeat 3 times.

- Often our tension conjures up images in our minds. Use your imagination productively to transform these images into something peaceful and positive. For example, if you are picturing tightly twisted ropes, imagine them slowly uncoiling and dancing for a snake charmer. Imagine tense red muscles, stretching, relaxing, and turning sky blue. Transform your fantasy of attacking your boss with a machete into an image of kneading a perfect loaf of bread and smell aromatic baking.

- Keep your head level and your body relaxed, and focus on a spot on the wall, with your eyes wide open. Count backwards from 5, closing your eyes a little as you go. By 3-2 they are nearly closed, by 1, your eyes are closed. Keep breathing slowly with your eyes closed and savor the relaxation.

- Affirmations are tried and true. Choose or invent your own: *"This too will pass so let go now."* *"Relax the jaw, lower the shoulders."* Etc.

5. Mindfulness

Mindfulness is a technique adapted from ancient Buddhist meditation practices. It has been successfully incorporated into innovative psychotherapies.

Mindfulness is a core component of Dialectical Behavior Therapy (DBT) and Mindfulness-Based Cognitive Therapy (MBCT). There is increasing research establishing that the mindfulness techniques learned from DBT and MBCT can help people with bipolar disorder regulate their moods.

What is mindfulness?

Mindfulness is all about being self-aware and staying in the present moment. It means paying attention to what is happening in the moment, in a non-judgmental way. It is focused and conscious attention to what is happening now, characterized by a spirit of openness and acceptance to what IS.

What does this have to do with bipolar disorder?

If we are fully living in the present moment, we cannot be rehashing the past, and beating ourselves up about what happened during our episodes of mania or depression.

If we are fully present, our thoughts are not racing or jumbled or foggy. We can experience the relief of being centered, calm, and relaxed – if only for a moment.

If we are fully present we are strengthening our mind in the way that exercise strengthens our muscles.

If we are fully present we experience less pain because we cannot do two things at once – to be mindfully engaged in any pleasurable activity means we cannot be thinking or feeling anything negative.

If we are fully present we are aware of our thoughts and feelings, and cannot impulsively or automatically "act out" destructive urges.

If we are fully present we get to truly know ourselves, establishing our own identity, and choosing our own direction in life.

If we are fully present we are immediately aware if we begin experiencing symptoms of mania or depression, and can get help before an episode fully develops.

Benefits of mindfulness for people with bipolar disorder

- Learn to control your thoughts
- Relaxation
- Improve concentration and memory
- Experience more positive emotions
- Control your behavior
- Get to know yourself
- Experience less pain, regret and shame
- Increased awareness of your symptoms
- Fewer and less serious episodes of depression and mania.

Mindfulness exercises

Traditionally, mindfulness is practiced through meditation. This was my introduction to mindfulness and it has been extremely helpful. However, it requires discipline and may be difficult without personal coaching and time to develop one's personal meditation practice. After I had been meditating for a while, I discovered that there are many mindfulness activities and exercises that are easier to "learn" than meditation. For example, today one of my favorite things to do is contemplative photography ("*miksang*"). The exercises below are all practical and intuitive ways to experience mindfulness. The key with all of them is to become completely engaged by focusing only and entirely on the activity:

- Mindfully walk by focusing on the feel of the ground as it connects with your foot in each and every step. Don't do anything else but walk and be in the moment – no talking, no iPod, no imaginary conversations or rehashing of past events. Feel the muscles in your legs move, and the sensation of the air and sun on your skin. Notice how you are breathing. Observe the colors and the shapes of the objects around you. Stay in the present and enjoy the moment.

Use this same approach and mindfully:

- Prepare or eat a meal

- Sit and breathe for one full minute as you watch the second hand turn on an old fashioned clock.

- Garden, clean, knit, paint your nails, fly a kite, play the piano, go to the park, do some yoga, pay bills – it doesn't matter what, but BE PRESENT!

Use the links below to discover more detailed descriptions of specific mindfulness exercises developed for the benefit of people with bipolar disorder.

Further resources

The Black Dog Institute, *Mindfulness in Everyday Life* at http://www.blackdoginstitute.org.au/docs/HandoutMindfulnessinEverydayLife.pdf

Sheri Van Dijk, *The Dialectical Behavior Therapy Skills Workbook for Bipolar Disorder*, New Harbinger, 2009 (use Google Books to read a preview)

6. Mood Charting

What is a bipolar mood chart?

A mood chart is a simple, patient driven tool that requires only a few minutes a day to complete. However, mood charts are extremely powerful and effective. This is because mood charts **provide a visual image** of how important pieces of information such as mood, medication, and life events all fit together.

Usually the mood chart contains space for at least the following information:

1. Date: there should be space for recording information for each day.

2. Mood scale: the scale would typically include a baseline which indicates feeling normal (no depression or mania) and then a range of points above the baseline for elevated mood, and below the baseline for depressed mood. A scale of -3 to +3 is common, but some charts have scales of -5 to +5 or even -10 to +10. I like to use -3 to +3.

3. How much sleep you got.

4. What medication was taken and the dosage.

5. Notes: this can be a record of life events considered relevant, such as stressors, therapy sessions, family gatherings, or notes about the workplace.

Other items that many people like to record include weight and any alcohol or drug use. Women often also include their menstrual cycle.

Someone who is experimenting with making diet and exercise changes may like to include that information.

(Feedback from folks following The Bipolar Diet shows that this is extremely helpful with managing medication related weight gain.)

I particularly like versions of mood charts that include columns for recording anxiety and irritability levels as both of these are issues for me.

The wonderful thing about mood charting is the exact contents can be customized for each person!

The example below is provided by NIMH (National Institute of Mental Health.) Don't worry if you can't read it all clearly – there is a link to full page versions of the chart you can download, along with the NIMH instructions: NIMH Daily Mood Chart

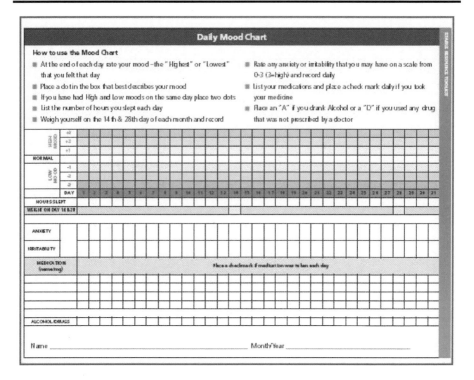

Why keep a mood chart?

PATTERN RECOGNITION: The mood chart for bipolar disorder is a visual tool that makes it much easier to identify patterns before serious problems develop. It is this pattern recognition that is my favorite part of mood charting. This may sound simple, but because there are so many factors involved (sleep, medication, life events, exercise, PMS) I find that charting is far easier, more effective and clearer than keeping a diary or simply trying to remember everything in between visits to the doctor.

OBJECTIVE EVIDENCE: I may suspect my fish oil is doing me good, or that my new medication is not as helpful as good old fashioned lithium, but I prefer collecting empirical data over a period of time to base my decisions on.

PRE-EMPTIVE STRIKES: The chart provides an early warning system that shows when my mood is becoming unstable. This makes it possible to make changes before I am caught in the middle of a major mood episode.

SELF AWARENESS: For me it is helpful to be aware of how I am feeling and of any ups and downs. It gives me a sense of control and makes me more sensitive to how my condition may be affecting my loved ones.

How to use bipolar mood charts

Each of the 3 versions included here comes with instructions. Here is a link to find all three. http://www.bipolar-lives.com/bipolar-mood-chart.html.

All you need to do is download a copy of the blank mood chart and then print it and make as many photocopies as you need.

1. NIMH Daily Mood Chart from the National Institute of Mental Health.
2. Mood Chart from the Massachusetts General Hospital Bipolar Clinic and Research Program.
3. Black Dog Institute Mood Chart.

These particular bipolar mood charts have been chosen to include in your toolkit because they are the professional versions that have been tested and validated, and are used and recognized by leading clinicians and researchers. Just choose the one that you like best.

Sharing your bipolar mood chart

Sharing charts for bipolar disorder with significant others, family, friends, therapists or medical professionals, or anyone else you consider part of your support network may be extremely helpful.

I like to share my chart for the following reasons:

1. Sometimes others are able to pick up patterns that I miss.

2. I want my spouse to feel informed, involved and trusted.

3. Sometimes my symptoms show up as an inclination to be secretive, paranoid and controlling - sharing my chart is the most effective way for me to short circuit this.

4. Knowledge is power, and I like power to be shared!

Bottom line . . .

By its very nature, the course of bipolar disorder is bumpy and unpredictable.

The whole point is that both the disorder and responses to treatment are likely to follow an irregular pattern that can be very confusing for the bipolar person and their care-givers.

The charts are a very easy but powerful tool to help everyone involved understand the relationships between the highs and lows of the disorder, possible stressors and triggers, the impact of medication, and the effectiveness of other measures such as diet and exercise.

Bonus 3: Bipolar Diet Glossary

Affective disorder: "Affect" is another word for mood.

Amino acid: The building blocks of protein. They are organic molecules consisting of nitrogen, carbon, oxygen, and hydrogen molecules. There are two kinds of amino acids: the essential amino acids that cannot be produced by our bodies and must be obtained from food, such as tyrosine, and the non-essential amino acids that can be produced by our body, although we may sometimes need supplementation, for example taurine.

Anticonvulsants: Drugs that relieve convulsions or seizures, primarily intended for the treatment of epilepsy. Some such as Depakote (valproate) are also effective for treating bipolar disorder, especially the manic phase.

Antidepressants: Drugs that relieve the symptoms of depression. For example, the SSRI Prozac.

Antipsychotics: Drugs that relieve the symptoms of psychosis. Some are now approved for the treatment of manic and psychotic symptoms in bipolar disorder. Abilify, Seroquel, Zyprexa, Geodan, and Risperdal are all examples of antipsychotics now used in the treatment of bipolar disorder.

Bipolar Disorder: Where the individual has episodes of mania (or hypomania) alone or with depressive episodes. Note that a person with bipolar disorder may only have experienced either mania or depression.

Bipolar I Disorder: Where a person has had at least one serious episode of mania that cannot be attributed to another cause such as substance abuse. Depressive episodes may have also occurred but are not a requirement for this diagnosis.

Bipolar II Disorder: Where a person has had at least one serious episode of depression that does not arise from another cause such as bereavement, and has also experienced some hypomania, but not full-blown mania or psychosis.

Bipolar Depression: Depression in a person with Bipolar Disorder. It may be contrasted with "unipolar depression" where the person only experiences depression and never has mood swings into hypomania or mania.

Bipolar NOS: The experience of hypomanic, manic, or depressive episodes that do not fit into any of the previously listed bipolar disorder categories.

CBT (Cognitive Behavioral Therapy): A psychotherapy, or "talk therapy" that focuses on identifying and changing thoughts and behaviors that may be maintaining symptoms or other negative consequences. Research indicates that this process of training the patient to think and act more positively is effective, and when combined with medication is more effective for treating bipolar disorder than medication alone.

Circadian Rhythm: The natural pattern of physiological and behavioral processes that are controlled by the "biological clock" or "body clock". These patterns of sleep-wake cycles, body temperature, blood pressure, and the release of hormones are usually timed to a 24 hour period. Evidence suggests that disturbances in a person's circadian rhythm can trigger bipolar mood episodes.

Clinical Depression: A chronic and persistent depression that is acute enough to require a clinical intervention from a mental health professional, for example psychiatric care or hospitalization.

Comorbidity: The coexistence of other illnesses or conditions that co-occur or exist simultaneously with the original diagnosed illness. Common comorbid conditions that affect people with bipolar disorder are substance abuse, thyroid malfunction, diabetes, anxiety and panic disorders, and obesity.

Cyclothymia: A milder form of bipolar disorder characterized by episodes of depression and hypomania that do not rise to the level of mania or major depression, but which do impact on the patient's life.

Delusion: A persistent false belief which is maintained by the believer despite evidence to the contrary or rational or logical proofs of why the belief must be mistaken.

Dopamine: Dopamine is an important neurotransmitter. It is a messenger formed in the brain and used by the central nervous system. It is involved in motor control, cognition, and perceptions of pleasure and reward. Abnormal dopamine levels occur in Parkinson's disease, paranoia, memory and concentration defect.

Double-blind, randomized, controlled clinical trial: the gold standard in research where research subjects are evenly divided into a group receiving the experimental intervention and a group receiving standard or no treatment. Neither the subjects nor the researchers (during the course of the study) know how subjects have been assigned. This practice reduces the chance for a "placebo effect," or clinical bias. The reason so few nutritional supplements can be conclusively said to help treat bipolar disorder is because of the lack of such trials for natural treatments. They are expensive to run and are usually only invested in by drug manufacturers seeking regulatory approval for proprietary drugs which may be patented in order to generate revenue.

DSM-IV: Diagnostic and Statistical Manual of Mental Disorders, Fourth Edition. This is the standard diagnostic text used by psychiatrists and published by the American Psychiatric Association. Mental Health Professionals use this manual when working with people in order to better understand their illness and potential treatment and to help third parties such as insurers understand the needs of the patient.

ECT (Electroconvulsive Therapy): Passing electric currents through the brain in order to cause a seizure, which in turn changes brain chemistry. It is an effective treatment for mood disorders and has manageable side effects, but is stigmatized due to early versions of the treatment which used stronger currents and caused more serious side effects.

Essential fatty acids (EFAs): These are the "good" fats such as the omega-3 found in fish oil. They cannot be created within the body and must be obtained from dietary sources. EFAs affect mood, behavior and inflammation, and there is persuasive research showing them to be very beneficial to people with bipolar disorder, particularly in treating depression.

Hallucinations: A distorted sensory perception such as hearing, seeing or sensing things that are not really there, although to the person experiencing it, the perception seems real.

Hypomania: This is lesser form of mania. The literal translation is "below mania". The hypomanic mood state is characterized by persistent and pervasive elevated or irritable mood, along with the thoughts and behaviors that express this interior state. It is distinguished from mania by the absence of psychotic symptoms and by its lower degree of impact on functioning. The DSM-IV distinguishes hypomania and mania in several ways. For example the duration of hypomania must be at least 4 days as opposed to 1 week for mania. Manic behavior is said to lead to negative consequences, whereas in hypomania there is the *potential* for painful consequences.

Mania: The DSM-IV defines mania, in the sense of bipolar mania, as: a distinct period of abnormally and persistently elevated, expansive, or irritable mood lasting at least one week (or less if hospitalization is necessary) and consisting of three or more of the following (four if the mood is irritable only):

- inflated self-esteem or grandiosity
- decreased need for sleep
- more talkative than usual or feeling pressure to keep talking
- racing thoughts or thoughts that seem to jump from topic to topic
- distractibility (e.g., attention is easily drawn to unimportant details)
- increased goal-directed activity
- excessive involvement in pleasurable activities that have a high potential for negative consequences (e.g., going on buying sprees, foolish business investments, promiscuous sex).

These symptoms must be severe enough to significantly impair the individual's functioning in work, school, or social relationships (or must require hospitalization or include psychotic features) and must not be due to the effects of a substance or general medical condition to qualify as a manic episode.

MAOIs (Monoamine Oxidase Inhibitors): Drugs that treat depression by blocking the enzyme 'monoamine oxidase' and thereby slowing the breakdown of certain neurotransmitters in the brain. Examples are Nardil and Parnate. It is very important to closely follow instructions on diet and drug interactions when taking MAOIs and obtain close medical supervision.

Mixed Episode: Mood episodes where the person experiences mania and depression at the same time. Mania during a mixed state often manifests as irritability or impulsivity.

Mood: A state of mind or emotions, as experienced by a person at a particular time.

Mood Disorder: Usually a specific psychiatric condition such as depression, mania, or one of the several forms of bipolar disorder. Traditionally the serious mood disorder of bipolar was referred to as manic-depressive illness.

Mood Stabilizer: A medication used to minimize the mood swings between depression and mania that characterize bipolar disorder. For example, lithium is a traditional mood stabilizer.

Neurotransmitter: A chemical substance, such as serotonin or dopamine, which transmits nerve impulses across a synapse.

Neuronutrient: Brain nutrients which provide essential nourishment to the brain, for example supplying all necessary building blocks for healthy functioning of neurotransmitters.

Norepinephrine: Both a hormone and a neurotransmitter. As a stress hormone it underlies the "flight or fight" response. Raising norepinephrine levels has been shown to treat depression, but also to induce mania.

Placebo: An inactive pill. This is sometimes called a "sugar pill." In some studies, participants may be assigned to take a placebo rather than the study medication.

Placebo effect: Sometimes people taking a study medication receive benefits that are not from the chemicals in the medicine. This is called a "placebo effect." For example, if a participant feels hopeful about a treatment, he or she may be more likely to notice positive changes than negatives ones. A researcher's hope may also sway a participant's response. Double-blind research design helps minimize the placebo effect.

Psychosis: A state of mental dysfunction where the individual loses touch with reality and often experiences hallucinations and/or delusions.

Psychotherapy: Non-physical or "talk" therapy between a therapist and client in order to address psychiatric or personality issues. There are many types of psychotherapy used to treat bipolar disorder. Research suggests that psychotherapy in combination with medication may be more effective than medication alone as a treatment for bipolar disorder.

Rapid Cycling: Four or more depressed or manic episodes per year.

Serotonin: A neurotransmitter with important functions, including control of appetite, mood and anger.

SNRI (Selective Noradrenaline Reuptake Inhibitors): Antidepressants such as Effexor, Pristiq and Cymbalta that selectively target the neurotransmitters norepinephrine AND serotonin in order to regulate mood. SSNIs work by inhibiting the uptake or re-absorption of both neurotransmitters, thus increasing the amounts available to the brain.

SSRI (Selective Serotonin Reuptake Inhibitors): Antidepressants such as Prozac, Lexapro and Zoloft that selectively target the neurotransmitter in order to regulate mood. SSRIs work by inhibiting the uptake or re-absorption of serotonin, thus increasing the amount available to the brain.

Stressor: A stressful situation occurring prior to a mood episode that may have triggered the mood swing into mania or depression.